DIAMONDS FOR RICE

DIAMONDS FOR RICE

Eric Evans

Matador
9 Priory Business Park,
Wistow Road, Kibworth Beauchamp,
Leicestershire. LE8 0RX
Tel: (+44) 116 279 2299
Fax: (+44) 116 279 2277
Email: books@troubador.co.uk
Web: www.troubador.co.uk/matador

ISBN 978 1785890 031

British Library Cataloguing in Publication Data.
A catalogue record for this book is available from the British Library.

Printed and bound by CPI Group (UK) Ltd, Croydon, CR0 4YY
Typeset in 11pt Aldine by Troubador Publishing Ltd, Leicester, UK

Matador is an imprint of Troubador Publishing Ltd

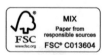

This book is dedicated to my daughters, Vicky and Louisa.

It is also dedicated to my bone marrow donor on two occasions, Axel Drewes. Axel calls me his genetic twin. He is my hero.

30% of the proceeds of this book will go to Anthony Nolan, Delete Blood Cancer UK and DKMS.

Introduction

By Anthony Nolan, who twice helped to save Eric's life

Every twenty minutes, someone in the UK finds out that they have blood cancer, like leukaemia. For many, a bone marrow transplant could be their only chance of survival – but only if they can find a matching donor. Thanks to the incredible legacy of a little boy called Anthony Nolan, there is hope. Anthony had a rare blood disorder and would only survive with a bone marrow donation from a stranger.

In the 1970s there was no system in place to find unrelated donors, but Anthony's dedicated mum Shirley didn't give up. Instead she did something amazing – she worked tirelessly to set up the world's first bone marrow register, so that Anthony and others like him would have the best chance of beating their illness.

Sadly, Anthony died before a matching donor could be found. But forty years on, thanks to his legacy, blood cancer charity Anthony Nolan is still going strong – and saving more lives than ever, by matching selfless people willing to donate their bone marrow to blood cancer patients in need of a transplant.

Since Shirley established the world's first bone marrow register, other countries have set up their own operations and there are now more than twenty-five million potential donors worldwide. Today, when someone needs a bone marrow or stem cell transplant, we search these combined registers to try to find a matching donor, breaking down international barriers in order to save lives.

We now help three people each day by finding that lifesaving match, curing thousands of people of blood cancers and other disorders.

To join the Anthony Nolan register, or support the charity's lifesaving work, go to www.anthonynolan.org. For more information please call 0303 303 0303.

Statement from DKMS

Statement from DKMS, who will promote the book throughout the world along with Anthony Nolan:

Launched in February 2013, Delete Blood Cancer UK is part of the DKMS (The Foundation for Donating Life) international network of charities that has already recruited over five million potential blood stem cell donors in Germany, Poland, Great Britain and the United States. This results in an average of thirty-four people donating their blood stem cells to patients in need each day.

With less than half of blood cancer patients in the UK finding the lifesaving match they need, our key mission is to increase the pool of potential donors. The aim is to find a suitable donor for every person in need of a blood stem cell donation.

The donor could be for a blood cancer or blood disorder patient in the UK or in another country. There are no borders when it comes to saving lives, as Axel and Eric have shown.

To find out more about the incredible work carried out by
Delete Blood Cancer UK, please visit
www.deletebloodcancer.org.uk
or call 020 8747 5620

My Mission

I traded bags of rice for diamonds. Little did the world's poorest children know, in a country ravaged by civil war, that those diamonds were to save my life. All around me there were murders, rapes and mutilations. I lost everything in that chaotic country. But I retained my love for the children who, without realising, saved me from the worst fate imaginable.

I can shed light on the turmoil in Liberia during the late Eighties. I was in the wrong place at the wrong time, with the wrong people, more than once during a savage conflict.

As if that wasn't enough, I stood next to the terrorist who bombed Orly airport and killed eight people. How did I survive that carnage?

As I lie in a hospital bed, awaiting my second bone marrow transplant, I reflect on six extraordinary decades. I left college at seventeen, profited from the North Sea Oil industry and became a millionaire at the age of twenty-eight. I owned a mansion, a fleet of luxury cars, two aircraft and a top nightclub. I cash-funded a consortium of treasure hunters, diving for Stalin's gold, lost on HMS Edinburgh after she was scuttled during World War Two.

I formed a unique friendship with the nephew of the James Bond author Ian Fleming, who has contributed to Diamonds for Rice. His rich family history is almost worth a book on its own.

There is a thirty per cent chance that I will die during the operation, but my story must be told and this book will be finished! I need to complete my work, which I started writing more than ten years ago at the time of my first transplant. I owe it all to my children, because I would like them to know everything about my life story. I could have died then, without them knowing anything about my life. The same applies now. My other reason for writing this book is to encourage potential donors to register with Anthony Nolan and Delete Blood Cancer.

The chemotherapy and first transplant took a lot out of me and now I must face it all again. Those millions I made in Liberia are a distant, but powerful memory; my logging company reaped huge rewards and collapsed like a pack of cards as Liberia erupted into civil war.

That spectacular country, riddled with corruption and soaked in blood, paved my life with gold – until I lost everything. Diamonds are certainly forever, and I keep thinking about those children who helped me to take the last flight out of the war-torn country. Scarlett's unique diamond, worth a small fortune and paid for with a bag of rice, eventually rescued me from that hell on earth. I survived brutal interrogations, but only just…

My outlook on life, and my values, changed completely when Scarlett and the other bush children gave me those diamonds. Ironically, the gems ensured my survival and the children may well have died in a bloodbath. They knew nothing about me or what I would do with the diamonds. They just wanted something to eat.

More traumas followed. I was diagnosed with Myelofibrosis, and that meant a long search for a bone marrow donor through the Anthony Nolan Register. I had that first successful transplant from a donor in Germany. I felt reborn. I became a founding member of the Full Circle Fund – a charity that supports patients with life-limiting illnesses at St George's Hospital in London.

Finally life was on the 'up' again – until the world economy imploded in 2008, my bone marrow disease returned shortly afterwards, and in January 2013 I declared myself bankrupt.

Since then my life has shrunk to enduring, happy fundamentals: my family, health and an appreciation of nature.

I read recently that life is not measured by the number of breaths we take, but by the number of moments that take our breath away.

My mind is still packed with the seeds of new adventures. I have to accept that any new escapades could never match the high drama contained in the following pages.

Who Wants To Be a Millionnaire?

'What do you want to be when you grow up?' my father asked at the tea table one night.

Gary, my brother who was eight at the time, replied: 'I want to be a doctor.'

'I want £1million, a gold Rolls Royce and my own number plate to match my initials – ESE 1,' I chipped in.

My father burst out laughing and switched the TV on. It was time for Emergency Ward 10, the nation's favourite programme in the late 1950s. Dad loved the show.

No other words were spoken that evening. My mum said nothing, and Dad kept chuckling.

I felt mortified, humiliated, and devastated. What was wrong with what I had said? I felt alone, as if on an island. I was saddened, at such a young age, that he saw my ambition as a joke. As he laughed, I became more determined to make my dream come true.

That day my father instilled in me the concrete desire to achieve my goals. At that time I did not know how or when. I was passionate and became even more driven.

That evening was a turning point. I was careful about what I said to him after that. My guard was up. I stayed intact on my island.

My ambition remained a driving force – even without the belief, enthusiasm and support of the one that I so much wanted to please.

As I dreamed on, five thousand miles away, deep in the

Liberian bush, generations of children endured primitive conditions without a penny to rub together. Yet they had diamonds to rub together. They knew where to find the most valuable gems in the world.

And what did they want for those diamonds? A few bags of rice.

Excerpt to make you smile

A large, loud, bleached blonde lady named Chantal joined us for dinner. She placed a napkin over her cleavage to collect any spillage and ate with gusto. She consumed pigs' trotters, tripe and other horrendous-looking side dishes as if her life depended on it.

Fat, grease and wine flew in all directions. I couldn't bear to watch as she sucked every last bone and splattered everyone on the table with debris. I took cover as the final remnants of her pig-sucking orgy whistled past my ear. She left the table, dripping with fatty residues, and still chewing on the tougher morsels. I have never seen a performance like that, anywhere on the planet, performed by man, woman or beast.

Her parting words filled me with dread as she plucked bits of trotter from her yellowing teeth: 'If you feel lonely tonight, my hotel door will be open.'

Excerpt to shock you

Boom! Bang! A burst of light stunned my eyes. I couldn't breathe. I had never seen such a bright light; I had never heard such a loud noise. As I stumbled around in the confusion, an eerie silence settled over the hall. A rush of air gave way to the sound of shattering glass, making another terrifying noise. My ears were numb; my brain was in a daze; my senses were transported to a different place. The normal hubbub of the airport terminal was replaced by a ghastly scene from a horror movie, all happening before my eyes in vivid colour and in agonising slow motion.

CHAPTER ONE

A Driving Force

June 25th – July 2nd 2014. St George's Hospital, London.

The isolation room is a comfortable size and, as I unpack and settle in, I feel cocooned – and in the safest of hands. By coincidence, I've been admitted back into the same room in St George's Hospital, where ten years ago, I had my first bone marrow (stem cell) transplant. Some of the staff are still here, which I find reassuring and demonstrates their knowledge and dedication.

Thankfully the first transplant was successful, and for many years I enjoyed the best of health, until symptoms of the disease – myelofibrosis – gradually reappeared.

Myelofibrosis – pronounced my-eh-lo-fy-bro-sis, is a rare blood disorder that causes scarring of the bone marrow; the soft inner part of our bones which produces blood cells. As the scar tissue develops in the bone marrow, it disrupts the body's normal production of red and white cells. The production of platelets, the mechanism to stop bleeding, is dealt a body blow.

As the illness progresses, fewer and fewer healthy blood cells are created; if left untreated a patient will die. I am extremely fortunate that the search for a donor for my first transplant eventually found someone in Germany who is not only an exact genetic match for me; he is also someone who generously offered to be there for me at any time in the future. The young man, Axel Drewes, has kept his word and is having twice daily injections into his stomach. These displace his bone marrow into his bloodstream, preparing his body for the harvesting of stem cells.

All of this is happening at a hospital in Dresden. I feel humbled and blessed by Axel's generosity.

Since this is my second bone marrow transplant there is a thirty per cent chance that I won't survive the procedure. But I'm calm and confident of a positive outcome and focus my attention on being among the other seventy per cent of that equation.

I sit on the bed and begin to reflect on my extraordinary life. All of my dramatic adventures come flooding back. I remember that, during a disastrous sea journey, my chances of survival appear to be much less than seventy per cent.

★★★

At the tender age of seventeen I applied for a clerical job in Great Yarmouth at a company called Offshore Marine, a subsidiary of Cunard.

I was offered the post at interview, with a starting salary of £315 a year, plus luncheon vouchers. It seemed like a small fortune in 1968 – as well as my first taste of freedom.

Although the job of shipping clerk didn't sound that exciting, I was determined to make the most of it. I knew it was a chance to broaden my horizons and one that I'd be a fool not to grasp. At the time, the exploration for gas and oil – or 'black gold' as the media called it – was just beginning in the North Sea.

The country was in economic crisis, with enormous pressure to get those natural resources flowing. Initial drilling had been unsuccessful, but in 1965 British Petroleum struck gas off the East Anglian coast. However, three months later on Boxing Day, the discovery was overshadowed when the rig, Sea Gem, capsized into the freezing cold waters of the North Sea with the loss of thirteen lives. However, drilling continued and in the ensuing years the industry and investment – as well as returns – grew rapidly. By the time I joined Offshore

Marine, during the autumn of 1968, it was certainly a well-established, flourishing company.

I arrived on a Monday morning and was shown to a desk groaning beneath the weight of six full paper trays. They completely blocked the view over the lively fishing wharf and Peg's Café. Soon, I would become one of their regular customers.

Offshore Marine's customers were oil companies that chartered supply vessels and who also required cargo-handling expertise, and/or the use of bonded warehouses. My work covered the record keeping for all of these areas, which needed to be accurately logged to satisfy HM Customs and Excise.

Filled with sudden energy, I'd cleared the trays in no time, much to the surprise of my new colleagues, Frank and Keith. They warned me over a cup of steaming tea and a chocolate Wagon Wheel at Peg's Cafe that, if I looked too ambitious, our boss would only give me more work to do. That was fine by me, I thought. After my disastrous school days, I was more than keen to feel some sense of achievement and maybe even the recognition that I craved so much.

I loved the sense of purpose and the pace of the place, and before long I was fully acquainted with all the regulations for vessels and cargo coming and going offshore. I was also taking driving lessons – paid for by Offshore Marine at £1.17/6d an hour in old money – and soon passed my test, which meant I could work evenings and weekends without relying on my dad for lifts. The feeling of freedom was exhilarating, and with every success my self-esteem grew. I also felt that, for the first time ever, I had real friends and was enjoying life.

Great Yarmouth Port was always active, and I never tired of watching the myriad of fishing boats and supply vessels entering the dock. I looked on in awe as they ventured back into the towering waves of the North Sea.[1] I longed for an opportunity to travel on one of the supply ships; as the control and regulation of passengers travelling to and from rigs was very relaxed in those days, arranging a trip on one of these vessels was fairly simple.

I secured a ride on the Suffolk Shore, a sixty-metre long supply ship that seemed enormous to my seventeen-year-old eyes. The last time I'd been on water was with my two brothers in a park during a holiday in Lowestoft, when I was aged eight. We'd huddled low in the back while our dad steered a set course in knee-high water at three miles an hour, and our mother sat, white-knuckled, clutching his arm in the front.

From the wheelhouse I watched the cranes loading the Suffolk Shore with five hundred tons of deck cargo, fuel and water for our intended destination – the Sedneth ll.

I had heard all about the monstrous, jack-up rig, towering above the sea. We also carried a hundred and fifty tons of sherbet yellow barytes, a mineral used in oil exploration. The round trip to the rig and back to Great Yarmouth would take several days. Perhaps it's a good thing that I had no idea what lay in store for me on the voyage. I had a foretaste of my fate as the Suffolk Shore pushed and pulled against the quay. Her massive hulk was buffeted by a gathering wind and a moving tide.

I watched intently as the crew lashed down the palletised deck cargo with heavy duty ropes and chains. The skies were a flat steel grey, foreboding to say the least, and a chill wind ripped through the harbour. We were released from the quay with a succession of violent movements to and fro. I saw the buildings on the shore from a different

1   I was still innocent about how vicious and violent the North Sea could be. Later that year, we received a call about a blow-out on an oil rig. A converted fishing vessel, the Hector Gannet, answered the distress call, struck the rig's leg in the tumultuous seas and capsized, killing three of the men on board.

perspective, high up in the wheelhouse, as I floated off into the unknown.

I gazed apprehensively ahead as the Suffolk Shore lurched forward into the churning, foaming waters. They loomed as far as the horizon and, I imagined, well beyond that. This, I reflected, was nothing like the boating park in Lowestoft with Mum and Dad; nor was there any way to get off, return to port and go home to tea, cake and Coronation Street.

Within half an hour the adventure I'd dreamed about had become a nightmare. Clearly, I'm not cut out to be a sailor, as I was feeling so sick by then that I was confined to my bunk. I clutched my stomach and tried not to actually vomit, although I soon failed to quell that urge. I had never felt so dreadful and full of despair.

Later on at tea the Captain, Len Gillings, said: 'It's only a mild swell. Force three going on four.'

I looked at him in disbelief before pushing away my tea and biscuits and bolting to the nearest toilet.

The weather was worsening by the hour, with the ship lurching ever more wildly from side to side and up and down. The waves appeared to me as frothing skyscrapers. We were sailing into a fierce wind, which I believed would seal my fate. I staggered around like a crab in a bucket. The Suffolk Shore bobbed continually between giant, ferocious waves like an abandoned ping pong ball. I was desperate to reach dry land – a rig, anything – because I felt that my time had come.

I found little solace that some of the crew were as sick as me. To my horror, the forecast on the radio announced that the storm would increase to force eight or nine. The cook's remedy was a hearty plate of bacon, eggs and beans. I was willing to try anything to feel better. I was spitting blood and had broken blood vessels in my cheeks. I found a corner of the galley where I wedged myself in and did my best with the greasy offering. I tried hard to pin down the highly mobile eggs as they slithered around the plate. Unfortunately, in my case, the cook was wrong and I was immediately sick again.

The wind continued to rise until it reached a tumultuous, rearing gale force twelve, the highest level on the wind-force scale. Even the captain was sick, though he had no option but to battle on against the sixty-foot waves. I hunkered down in my cabin for the duration. Through a porthole all I could see, when I managed to lift my head from the bunk, was rain hurled from the sky as the ship rose endlessly on the crest of the swell.

Then an abyss of water represented the gateway to hell as the ship and its vulnerable human cargo plunged back down over a watery precipice.

The sea was roaring; its mood was terrifying. The propellers, clean out of the water on the crest of the mighty waves, whined their protest at the onslaught. The hull shuddered as it plunged down into each trough before rising, creaking and groaning, on the next crest. By then the deck was awash with seawater and the cargo pitched dangerously, tugging at its web of ropes and steel chains. Gradually, one by one, the securing mesh disintegrated under the worst pounding nature could provide. The pallets slid along the deck and disappeared off the back of the boat into the abyss. Five hundred tons of cargo, lost from one ship in one storm. I could scarcely believe it.

My nightmare of all nightmares persisted for thirty-six hours. I doubted whether the ship, crew or this distressed passenger would survive. Eventually, as day darkened into night, the storm eased, and the sea gradually subsided.

I strained to see a dot on the horizon. It was a mere speck, yet it grew and grew into a colossus. As dawn broke and a strong sun emerged over the horizon, the Suffolk Shore was dwarfed by the Sedneth ll, towering several hundred feet above sea level.

Finally, we were safe. The storm died down completely, just as quickly as it had erupted. We had no deck cargo left to deliver apart from the contents of tanks down below, holding water and chemicals for the rig.

As we headed back to Great Yarmouth, the wind dropped completely. A full moon lit up the calm seas and followed us until daybreak. I counted the stars and concluded that they were all lucky ones for me.

It was truly beautiful. I spent all night in the wheelhouse enjoying the seascape and, finally, some food.

The return voyage could not make up for my near-death experience. I vowed never to set foot on a boat again.

I found it hard to believe that I was still alive.

CHAPTER TWO

In Search of Black Gold

June 25ᵗʰ – July 2ⁿᵈ 2014. Treatment continues at St George's Hospital, London.

As I unpack I feel a calm settle over me. Although I am in an isolation suite I do not feel alone and my previous experience tells me I'm in the best possible hands. It's not long before I'm given two units of blood, since my blood count is so low, and two nebulisers[2] with medication to protect my lungs and airways. My immune system is so low that I would not be able to fight any infections at the moment.

The Hickman Line is inserted with local anaesthetic. This line is a catheter, inserted under sedation into the central venous system for the long-term administration of medications.

By then it's 3.30 p.m. and I'm sent for an X-ray to check that the line is in place. Unfortunately the X-ray shows that it is too far in, so the doctor will have to review this and possibly pull it back up. My chemotherapy is due to begin tomorrow, and I'm worried about a pain in my left kidney.

I tell the haematologist in the isolation unit about the pain and ask if it might be a stone, since I had renal colic twice in my twenties and am familiar with the horrific pain. I am told it is one of the worst pains you can have – I confirm this is correct.

I'm taken for a further X-ray, though no stone is revealed. The

2   A nebuliser pushes compressed air through liquid medication, which makes it into a mist that is then inhaled through a mouthpiece. It is the best way to introduce medication into the lungs.

specialist decides I need to have a CAT scan later that evening and, if there is a kidney stone, removal will be necessary and the bone marrow transplant delayed.

Of course I don't want that delay, but I have little choice in the matter. I must embrace whatever I'm delivered. The CAT scan unit is open 24 hours a day in St George's. A porter arrives just after midnight to wheel me down for an unequivocal determination on whether there is, in fact, a kidney stone.

The department is surprisingly busy, but I'm soon X-rayed and returned to my room. With my mind stumbling through the events of the day I ask for, and am given, a sleeping pill. I'm about to take it when a urologist comes in and tells me that I have a kidney stone blocking a tract on my left side, and two stones on my right. They are most concerned about the one on my left, which they say must be dealt with immediately; the oncologist, I am told, will discuss it all with me in the morning.

With that I take my pill and fall asleep…and I drift back to those early days as a teenager, trying to make my mark in the world.

★★★

The only silver lining I could salvage from the Suffolk Shore near-death event was its value as an anecdote. As an inexperienced seventeen-year-old, I recognised the value of my brave feat on the high seas. What a story to tell the girls.

I was also determined to have my first drink of alcohol as, beyond the odd lager and lemonade with my dad, I hadn't yet tasted any booze.

That New Year's Eve, in 1968, I hit the high spots of Great Yarmouth with three colleagues from the office, hoping to redress both of those points. I was in the mood to celebrate, having just been given a £50 end of year bonus by Offshore Marine. We began the evening at a pub where I followed the lead of my friend who'd ordered a pint of bitter.

For someone who hadn't drunk alcohol before, the glass looked enormous and the dark liquid inside appeared to be daunting. I took my first sip and knew immediately that the taste of the drink was not for me, but I had no choice other than to persevere – or else I'd never live it down. The drink at least gave me a bit of Dutch courage and I managed a tentative flirt with an attractive blonde who was sitting nearby.

My confidence soared. Suddenly, with a drink in my hand, some money in my pocket and a smile from a girl, I was a man of the world! I wanted everything; I wanted success on a grand scale.

I struggled to the bottom of my glass.

'The same again, Eric?' asked my friend.

'Thanks,' I replied, trying not to look reluctant.

The pub was filling up and my spirits rose with the volume. This was definitely the best night of my life so far.

But the fun didn't stop there. Five pubs, six and a half pints, and several packets of crisps later, we ended up in the Tower Ballroom on the Great Yarmouth seafront. This was a whole new world for me. The vast room glittered. A live band played the latest hits from Diana Ross and The Supremes, Johnny Nash and The Doors. Dazzling couples shimmered and shimmied around the ballroom; the women were dressed in a rainbow of colours.

Suddenly the colours, the music and the whirling figures were spinning out of control in my head. An acoustic kaleidoscope was attempting to ensnare me in its psychedelic maze. By now, it was close to midnight.

I leaned against one of the pillars. I thought a glass of water would help, but I knew that the others would never let me forget it. Instead I was determined to focus on the band at the far end, and not the rollercoaster of blurred images all around me. I felt dizzy. As midnight struck I was fleeing like Cinderella out of the ballroom – though in my case it was not back home but to the toilet, where I slid to the floor, gripped the porcelain and vomited repeatedly. It was like being back on the Suffolk Shore all over again. And, as I'd vowed never to go back to sea after that adventure, this time I swore myself off that horrible beer.

★★★

In 1969, there was another significant event for the world, apart from the moon landing. The first major discoveries of oil were made in the North Sea, beginning with the find at Ekofisk and then the Montrose Field. At the same time my efforts also paid off and I was transferred at the age of eighteen by Offshore Marine to Heysham Port, near Morecombe Bay on the northwest coast of England. The port was being used as a base by Gulf Oil and the Gas Council to explore beneath the Irish Sea.

Until then, my travels had not extended beyond the journey to boarding school in Wolverhampton, or our holidays along the east coast for our annual break when Dad had taken a whole day – and at least three long stops to relieve the stress – to drive a hundred or so miles.

My new job was overseeing the stock control and Customs and Excise records as well as all the logistics for Gulf Oil supply vessels. The American giant was using Offshore Marine's know-how and facilities to assist their drilling operations. With the promotion came my own vehicle – a Morris 1000 van.

As my family lined up to wave me off from Lowestoft, I felt not only a surge of excitement, but also the first true freedom in my life. I was heading off on my own three hundred miles away to the northwest coast and, for the first time ever, on a motorway.

Despite my modest salary of six pounds and five shillings a week, before deductions, plus the perks of a van, petrol, hotel and board, I felt as though I had the world at my feet. It seemed as if I had infinite opportunities in front of me, and I was determined to make the most of them. I made the journey in five hours, stopping only once for petrol; what a contrast to my tortuous travels to the seaside, huddled in the back of the car behind Mum and Dad.

Morecombe Bay was a popular resort town in 1969 – famous in those days for the Miss UK contest. You could see the mountains of the nearby Lake District, while the town itself was smart and self-assured. Offshore Marine booked me into the Grosvenor Hotel. It was a tall, cumbersome, red brick Victorian building with sixty rooms that sat clumsily astride the promenade. The hotel had views of the sea and the bay. For the next eight and a half months, it was to be my home from home.

Before long I was happily settled in and getting to know the staff. There were around twenty or so people working at the hotel, but one girl really stood out. I just couldn't get her out of my head. Frances Cairns was working at the hotel as a chambermaid while training to be a teacher at Charlotte Mason College in Ambleside. She was two years older than me and had cornflower blue eyes with a playful sparkle that I found particularly attractive, a warm smile, and dark brown hair. But, more importantly, she liked me. Eventually, I plucked up the courage to ask her out – this being the first time I'd actively pursued a girl – and we began dating.

Generally we hung out in the cosy basement Cellar Café in Morecambe, enjoying their wonderfully rich coffee and home-made apple pie, and chatting. We both came from backgrounds that had hemmed us in and kept us innocent of the wider world. For us, this new-found freedom was dazzling. We shared a zest for life and a desire, if not for adventure, then at least to explore the planet.

We had ambition and determination in common, and that drew us together. I loved the fact that Frances wanted to be a teacher, and that she was paying her own way to achieve her goal. I also loved her mix of innocence and vitality. We soon found that we were spending more and more time together, and eventually we ended up in my rickety single bed in my hotel room – number 19 – on a cold evening in early December. With no expectations or condoms – just the sound of the howling wind and the waves careering over the pier – we found first love.

Our passions continued to run unchecked for the next few months, until Frances broke the news that she was pregnant. My naivety was such that it came as an enormous shock. I managed to remain fairly calm, under the circumstances, and pondered over the best way to tell my parents. A public appearance would settle the matter rather than hiding at the end of a telephone, I decided.

'You're both far too young to get married; it would be a mistake,' said my mother on the evening I broke the news. 'You're under no obligation to Frances – you can always get rid of the baby.'

She also warned me that she would never welcome Frances into our family home, or look after the child. I had never heard her sounding so harsh. She put me back on that island, where my dad had placed me unceremoniously over a decade ago.

'Dad?' I asked, turning to the disinterested figure in the armchair. But my father simply shrugged and carried on watching television as he always did.

Obviously my mum's judgement was clouded by her own experience. She'd never talked about her days as a ballerina with us, but clearly she knew only too well how a pregnancy could irrevocably change the course of someone's life. She could envisage me reliving her own experiences and her many regrets.

Despite deep reservations from both sets of parents, Frances and I were married at Kendal Town Hall's Registry

Office on 21 March 1970, nineteen days after my nineteenth birthday. Frances wore a blue mini dress with a Peter Pan collar and a red Alice band, and I had on a brand new £7 rust-coloured herringbone made-to-measure suit. I knew that I was not ready to be married, but I had a child coming and I was in love. I was happy to give Frances a £50 diamond ring, after saving up, and make the commitment. That was ten times my weekly net wage.

We spent our wedding night at the Strathmore Hotel on the East Promenade in Morecombe, but were forced to part a few days later while Frances finished her teacher training. I returned to my work as a shipping clerk in Great Yarmouth, although I drove to Ambleside most weekends, blasting out Glen Campbell's Galveston as I drove. That wasn't the last I was to hear of Glen!

I looked around for a suitable home to house my wife and future baby. I found a drab, grey two-roomed flat to rent for £30 a month on Kirkley Cliff in Lowestoft. It was basic, but all I could afford.

When Frances qualified as a teacher I drove to collect her from the college in Ambleside in my 1956 jet black 1500 Wolseley, which we'd bought for £50. We loaded the car and drove back on a Sunday afternoon. Just outside Preston on the newly-built M6, I heard the unmistakable sound of rupturing metal from the engine.

My pride and joy ground to a halt. Eventually we were towed to a car auction site where we found out that the big end had blown and my one asset in the world was now almost worthless. We watched the car being sold for £8 and 10 shillings and then thumbed our way forlornly back to Lowestoft, arriving late that night. It was not an auspicious start to our married life together.

We now had no car and little money. It was time for me to make some extra cash, just to survive. I happily did every call-out to the docks in the evenings or at weekends in Great Yarmouth, not only to get the overtime pay, but also use of the company vehicle. Frances' mother, Jessie, arrived to stay until the birth and I was banished from the bedroom to a borrowed camp bed. Jessie was a strong, difficult woman – all in all, it was not an easy time for me.

However, the happy outcome of this period was that, on 22 August 1970, with Frances hollering and me being relegated by the doctor to stalk the corridor in the time-honoured tradition of anxious husbands, we became parents to Vicky. My world was changed in an instant. One glimpse of her tiny, fragile face and I knew that I was ready to assume the responsibility of being a father.

Jessie decided to stay on for a while after the birth to help Frances, and they passed the time either at home or on the promenade. It was something of a relief when Jessie returned home to Ramsbottom a few weeks later.

Frances' mother loaned us £150 as the deposit on a brand new bungalow costing £3,300 in Rollesby, a small village not far from Great Yarmouth. To this day, I have no idea why my father advised us against buying a property – anyway, I took no notice.

Proud and excited, and certain that we were making the right decision, we moved into our own home in February 1972, and at the same time I bought a second-hand Austin A40 for £140.

Frances was working as a supply teacher at a local school in Great Yarmouth and my reputation at Offshore Marine had been greatly boosted after my stint at Heysham Port. I felt vindicated. All the doubters had questioned my ability to look after Frances and our baby daughter Vicky, yet we were doing more than fine; we were thriving.

One day I was called into the manager's office and asked if I would go to Aberdeen to sort out some serious problems for a client. Of course, I agreed to go. I arrived in the city of Aberdeen at the height of summer. Once there it wasn't long before I resolved the situation with HM Customs and Excise. The government regulators were fairly new to the oil industry and, at the age of twenty, I was regarded as an expert!

I made my mark with all involved in the industry. Shortly after my return to Great Yarmouth I was offered a promotion with a permanent move to Aberdeen.

Frances had never liked me going away, and was certainly not at all happy at the thought of us moving. She'd had a difficult upbringing, living in a two-up two-down house with an outside toilet, and from that difficult start had eventually qualified as a teacher. My dreams of becoming a millionaire were still just that: dreams.

'We have a nice house and we should be thankful for that,' Frances scolded. 'We are comfortable enough. We've got a nice car and a good lifestyle. Why don't we just enjoy what we have?'

Her ambitions had been realised. Done and dusted. She had peaked. My ambitions were only just beginning to find their form. I could see the opportunities opening up in Aberdeen, as oil exploration took over the city, and I was determined to accept the promotion.

Eventually Frances agreed to the move. While we were going through the process of selling our home in Rollesby and buying a new one, I stayed in a hotel in Aberdeen during the week. My trusty Austin had been replaced by a snazzy Ford Cortina. I drove home in my silver machine to be with my family at weekends – a journey of over five hundred miles each way.

Thankfully, before long we'd sold our recently bought bungalow and purchased a detached house for £6,110 in Findon, a quaint fishing village just south of Aberdeen. Shortly after we'd moved there, as a gesture of appeasement, I bought Frances a shaggy Pyrenean Mountain dog. We named him Arran.

An unexpected thrill in the Granite City was the phenomenon known as Aurora Borealis or the 'Northern Lights of Old Aberdeen' in the famous song. This brilliant natural light display in the sky is a feature of the Arctic and Antarctic. I stood, transfixed at the dockside while a myriad of colours lit up the sky.

My next mission was to take me far beyond those Northern Lights as I attempted to make a dazzling impression on the other side of the pond.

CHAPTER THREE

From Aberdeen To Texas

Kidney stone treatment continues at St George's Hospital.

I wake at 7 a.m. and lie on my bed thinking about the latest turn in my medical saga, until I get up an hour later to shower and dress. The urologist arrives and confirms that they will insert a stent – a short mesh tube – into each kidney so they can function normally despite the stones. They will perform that operation tomorrow, and the bone marrow transplant will be postponed until one particularly dangerous stone has gone. I resolve to begin drinking copious amounts of water to hopefully resolve the matter naturally.

From there the day unfolds in a rapid succession of being given units of blood and pills – anti-sickness and antibiotics – having the Hickman Line in my chest pulled up (which hurt more than I care to admit), and then having morphine for the pain in my kidney. My brother Gary, a retired Ear, Nose and Throat Surgeon, is concerned about the latest development. I tell him that problems with the stone during the bone marrow transplant could have serious consequences.

The rest of the day and evening pass fairly quickly, with an X-ray to check that the Hickman Line is now in place. I have an early light meal, listen to music and watch the football. The pain from the kidney stone kicks in again and I'm given more morphine and a sleeping pill. In my mind, I live the American dream…

★★★

Work in Aberdeen was exciting and challenging. Offshore Marine had several contracts with oil companies – all requiring constant attention. It was decided that I would look after Hamilton Brothers Oil and Gas, a long established and very successful privately owned company headquartered in Denver, Colorado. They'd hired the drill ship Glomar 3 from Global Marine to begin exploration in the North Sea, using Aberdeen as the base.

Hamilton Brothers and Global Marine sent operational staff to Aberdeen from America. I dealt with Jack Pillow at Hamilton Oil[3] and Bobby Billups at Global.

Jack was a loud, hard-living, middle-aged, Bourbon-drinking, steak eating, cigar smoking, tobacco chewing, rough and tough Texan. He was counterbalanced in business by his quiet and smartly dressed right-hand man, Ron Manery.

In addition their staff included Doyle Bray, who ran their back office and had responsibility for paying accounts and, through me, organising the logistics of people and equipment to and from the drill ship. On board, responsible for the drilling operation, Hamilton employed another rough Texan called Herbert Becker. I can clearly picture him savagely trimming his nails with a penknife in the office one day.

Herbert and Jack were in constant communication by radio and telex; Jack in our frantic office and Herbert wallowing around at sea on the Glomar 3.

Jack Pillow had a tough reputation and you wouldn't want to cross him or provide him with bad service. Certainly to begin with, I knew I had to give attention to every detail. Fred and Ferris Hamilton, who had started the company in 1950, building it from the ground up, ran the head office in Denver and relied on Jack to control operations in Aberdeen.

---

3   Fred Hamilton has been awarded 2014 Citizen of the West in the US, to honour his achievements as a pioneer in the energy industry and benefactor for the arts

Hamilton Brothers' office was in Rubislaw Terrace, a smart road in the city close to the Marcliffe Hotel, where Jack and Ron stayed and ventured back and forth for breakfast, lunch and dinner.

The office was always busy as they drilled 24/7: day flowed into night with Jack constantly on the radio to the drill ship and its owners, or on the phone to Denver. And it was my job to ensure that the drill ship's supply needs were met at all times. Vessels had to be loaded and unloaded at a moment's notice.

The company had several supply vessels on hire, plus two helicopters on charter from Bristows at my disposal. But to complicate matters the Glomar 3, being a drill ship, was not suited for the North Sea weather and kept breaking away from more than a hundred tons of anchors. This entailed having her towed back to the drilling location on many occasions.

Every day in the office was frantic. Jack sat behind his desk, like a tornado of energy, smoking a cigar or chewing tobacco. He was able to spit from his desk and successfully hurl the swirling black sludge into the waste bin twenty feet away, and in fact he was expert at this. He did miss occasionally, leaving an indelible stain on the walls. He'd had a lot of practice, as the cleaner would testify. Actually Jack married her, and so I imagine that this spitting routine lasted well into their married life.

Jack was certainly larger than life – and with a commanding presence. If things went wrong you'd certainly know about it. If suppliers failed to deliver he'd give them the roasting of their lives, to say the least.

Hamilton Brothers appeared to have unlimited funds and rented wherever possible – from the drill ship to the cars, and supply boats to office desks – in case they needed to leave a barren location. They were a pioneering company and led the way in using a floating drilling and production platform, which Ferris Hamilton later designed and then had built to survive conditions in the North Sea.

In August 1971 Hamilton Brothers discovered large oil reserves in Block 30/24 of the United Kingdom Continental Shelf, a hundred and ninety miles southeast of Aberdeen. The find was confirmed the following year and the area became known as the Argyll Field.

After Hamilton Brothers found oil, Glomar 3 was brought into port to be discharged of all hired equipment. I was responsible for ensuring that everything was 'off hire' as soon as possible. The drill ship looked like a tiny dot in the North Sea; in port it dominated the skyline and even made the front page of the Aberdeen Press and Journal. Crowds came down to see her tied up on the city's centre quay.

Jack said that it would take me two or possibly three days to discharge everything off the drill ship. However, I was more than prepared when she arrived in port, having three gangs of dockers, three cranes and dozens of trucks on standby. We completed the task in thirty-six hours.

At that point my life became even busier. Having made their first oil discovery in the Argyll field, Hamilton Brothers then progressed into oil production. The company must have been more than satisfied with the service I'd given them, as they asked me to become their first UK employee. My second ever job was with an American oil company. I wouldn't have felt out of place in the cast of Dallas.

As Hamilton's logistics manager it was my job to organise whatever supplies and equipment were needed on their rigs. I was on call literally all hours – day, night, weekends, birthdays and even Christmas and New Year, if necessary.

The expense involved in running the rigs was astronomical. Supply vessels and helicopters operated twenty-four hours a day between Aberdeen and the rigs. And again Hamilton Brothers were leading the way in the industry, being the first company to produce oil from a short buoy mooring, loading offshore directly into oil tankers.

Jack Pillow was now my boss and, while he appeared to be a hard taskmaster, I soon discovered that – beneath the enamel – lay a soft centre. He always treated me well, giving me the same privileges as their long-term employees. He ensured that I drove a top-of-the range Vauxhall – the same car driven by key personnel. This transpired after Doyle hired the smallest possible car for me to drive, and Jack was obviously unimpressed.

I turned twenty-one, celebrating the occasion with a party at home in Findon. On 25 June I watched my second daughter, Louisa, being born at the Fonthill Maternity Unit in Aberdeen. She had her mother's blue eyes and feathery dark hair. As I'd missed Vicky's birth, seeing Louisa come into the world was a lifetime highlight for me. I certainly felt that, aged twenty-one, I had it all – a fantastic family, superb home life and a key job in the oil industry.

That year Frances and I found a deserted 'steading' – an old Scottish farmhouse – further down the coast in the former fishing village of Crawton, south of Aberdeen. The farm stood isolated on an incline at the head of a valley and had impressive sea views with a stream flowing over the cliffs. Although the location was a fair distance from Aberdeen, the property oozed potential. We paid £3,100 in 1973 and began converting the buildings into a home.

It took six months to make the place habitable – and even when we moved in, there was no front door. It was perfect for our young daughters. Arran, our Pyrenean dog, loved the place. He proved to be a proficient rat-catcher, killing the vermin with a single swipe of his paw! The isolated farmhouse was the ideal venue for parties forty odd years ago. We belted out music around the hillside; our favourites were Don McLean's 'American Pie', 'The Air That We Breathe' by the Hollies, and

Charlie Rich's song about the most beautiful girl in the world. American Pie was a foretaste of things to come.

Frances began taking driving lessons and soon passed her test. On the one hand she seemed to be settling into the area, while on the other she talked about returning to Morecombe Bay to buy and run a guest house.

It was a conversation that I skirted around, too afraid to tell her that, in my mind, it would never happen; perhaps I was upset that she didn't appreciate how much I was achieving.

The following year Hamilton Brothers asked me to travel to Freeport, a town in Texas about an hour from Houston on the Gulf of Mexico. They wanted me to run the shore-based logistics for a jack-up rig fifteen miles into the gulf. The whole team from Aberdeen were going, except for Doyle, who was to take care of the Aberdeen office in our absence.

Having never been abroad, I was incredibly excited at the prospect; however, Frances was furious. The cracks in our marriage were becoming like chasms. There was no way I could refuse the offer from Hamilton Brothers; they were my employers.

After a terrible row with Frances, I boarded my first ever flight, travelling first class on a British Caledonian DC 10 from Prestwick to Houston. I was joined on the plane by Al Purvis, the Hamilton Oil 'mud man' who was tall, quiet and handsome. He oversaw the down-hole mud mix and inspected the core samples of earth. For me, it was quite an introduction to flying with champagne and brilliant food all the way.

I remember the blast of heat and humidity as we left the airport terminal in Houston, which left me feeling as though my lips and nose were burning. This was my first experience of high humidity – quite a shock to the system.

We took a taxi to The Houston Oaks, a luxury hotel attached to a vast, upmarket shopping mall called The Galleria. The complex, with a massive ice rink in the centre, was spectacular. That evening we all met at the hotel for dinner and I felt thrilled that, aged twenty-two, I was sitting there with all these old Texan oil hands.

Early the following morning we drove down to the Holiday Inn in Freeport – our intended home for the next six months. Frances and the girls were hoping to join me after four weeks.

From there we headed to the docks where I instantly settled into my portable office. Most of the equipment was there already, with the supply vessel due to arrive that morning. Just like clockwork we all fitted into our respective roles. The rig confirmed that it would be on location and ready to start drilling, and so I dispatched the first vessel with the start-up supplies. The routine was exactly the same as in Aberdeen – just a different location.

I used to eat mostly with the guys at the hotel, although sometimes we'd go out to a restaurant and occasionally Jack and I would sit together at the hotel bar. One evening I decided to venture out and asked the hotel clerk to recommend a typically Texan venue for me to visit. I drove fifteen miles down the road in my Oldsmobile hire car and pulled up at a bar.

Outside there were mostly colourful 4x4s. Inside, I was welcomed with the Eagles classic, Hotel California, shuddering out of a battered, gigantic loudspeaker. The assembled gathering in jeans, cowboy boots and Stetson hats turned around to study me. I must have looked out of place in my slacks, shirt and jacket. I hardly looked like an everyday Texan!

Next on the playlist, Glen Campbell belted out Wichita Lineman from the quivering speaker. I walked up to the bar, ordered a bottle of beer and began chatting to everyone.

I was able to discuss Charlie Rich's 'beautiful girl in the world' number and describe how it had been my favourite at Scottish parties. I had a great night and banked another wonderful memory.

During that 1973 trip I also had my first taste of McDonalds – but this was nothing like the UK version of today. This outlet in Freeport served up sensational giant burgers with a choice of tasty, fresh salads and dressings. Was it really a McDonald's?

Jack also taught me where snakes were most likely to sleep and how to avoid them. One day his car suddenly swerved violently across the road. I thought he'd had some sort of seizure.

'Rattlesnake,' he muttered. 'They're deadly, so we need to kill them before they get us.'

Jack's office was like a sauna, despite the air conditioning. He sent me off to the nearby store to buy an ice-cold watermelon. I duly set off to complete the task, but couldn't tell the difference between a pumpkin and a watermelon. I returned with a pumpkin, much to the amusement of Jack who couldn't stop laughing and told the story repeatedly, in hysterics.

One Sunday Jack and I drove the forty-five miles up to Galveston, a city that held a certain romance with me because of that song made famous by Glen Campbell. By this time Jack was becoming much more relaxed. He opened up about his personal life and described how he'd come up through the ranks of the oil industry. It was evident that he was both experienced and enthusiastic about the business; but then as the Hamilton Brothers' key man, he would have to be. He had multi-million dollars of spending power under his control. The figures were truly massive.

Galveston, when we arrived there, was a typical seaside resort with a promenade, pier, and an endless sandy beach stretching deep into the distance. The place was known, fondly, throughout the world. I almost had to pinch myself that I was there for a Sunday lunch of freshly caught lobster.

I could still imagine Galveston's sea winds blowin' when I arrived back in Freeport. The peace was shattered, though, when a frantic Jack phoned my room at two in the morning.

'Eric, we've got a problem with the rig. We need to get down to the docks now. We may need to load a boat immediately.'

I dressed quickly and drove to the docks in a hurry. When I arrived, Jack told me that a leg on the jack-up rig had plunged into a softer pocket on the sea bed and then buckled. The rig was listing dangerously, so we dispatched helicopters to evacuate all but essential crew. We had hoped to right the position, but the damage was too severe so we had to close down the operation.

Jack said that I should call when I'd tied up all the loose ends in Freeport. I could see why the company rented everything, instead of buying, because they could move on seamlessly. Jack invited me to Hamilton Oil's headquarters in Denver, Colorado. So I spent the next ten days winding down the shore operation and collecting all the accounts in preparation for travelling to Denver. I said that I would drive to San Antonio, to take in some scenery, and fly from there instead of Houston.

I left the hotel in Freeport and set out on the unknown Texas roads for what seemed like a great adventure.

The road network in 1973 bore no resemblance to the America of today. I remember driving on normal roads, not freeways, and stopping off for a break after a hundred or so miles at a shack-type cafe. By then I'd got used to being stared at when I ordered a coke and a sandwich. Kenny Rogers urged Ruby not to go to town, while John Denver extolled the virtues of West Virginia's country roads. And, just to make me feel at home on the American seaside, the Wurlitzer juke box gave regular renditions of Surfin' USA by the Beach Boys.

For the next couple of days I became a tourist and had an amazing time. I visited the site of the Alamo; I was surprised that it was such a small ruin. Nevertheless it was fascinating to see the site of the famous battle in the Texas Revolution. I was also struck by the number of beggars on the streets. What a contrast to my world in Aberdeen.

I managed to get a window seat on the flight to Denver and was excited to be heading to yet another new destination. However, on arrival at the airport, a mile above sea level, I experienced the worst nose bleed I could remember. Thankfully, by the time I'd collected my luggage, it had subsided and I headed directly to Hamilton Oil's headquarters – the entire top floor of a high-rise block in the business district.

'Hi, you must be Eric,' the attractive, smartly-dressed receptionist greeted me, dispelling my nerves immediately. 'We're all pleased to see you here. We've all heard about you from Jack and Ron.'

Looking up from her face, I could see the vast sweep of the Rocky Mountains through the windows behind her, stretching across the horizon and soaring to the sky. I was transfixed with the view, and would have happily soaked it in for a while but Ron, Jack and Al had heard of my arrival and soon swarmed around me. They were keen to show off the sumptuous offices and introduce me to the company's owners.

Both Fred and Ferris Hamilton were straight out of the James Stewart mould – tall and elegant, with an easy-going charm. They thanked me for my work so far with the company in Aberdeen and the Gulf as we sat down for coffee. They said they'd reserved a room for me in a hotel close by, and I should check in, relax, and drive up into the Rocky Mountains. They even provided a hire car. At the age of twenty-two, I felt like a fully-fledged executive.

The next morning I was up early, eager to explore the famed mountains. Denver is a mile above sea level, yet the mountains rose even further into the sky and clouds. As I drove through a park and higher into the mountain passes I was conscious of my raised heartbeat in the thinning air. It was the fall. The aspen trees had turned a vibrant yellow and hot orange before shedding their leaves. It was a dirt road, too; if the Lone Ranger and Tonto passed by on their horses, being chased by American Indians, I wouldn't have been surprised.

I parked next to a church, perched in the mountains. Just walking made me breathless, although I had planned to climb the steps to the top of the church tower. I made it to the church, but could go no further: I was light-headed and felt sick because of the lack of oxygen, so I drove quickly back down the mountain to regain my senses.

That evening, Ron picked me up at the hotel and drove me to a classy restaurant down town. Jack and Al were all waiting eagerly for us. Dinner was superb, and the evening was filled with tales of oil exploits in America. I sat transfixed to learn about the adventures of these old Texan hands.

The following day I returned to the office to settle all the financial matters from the Freeport operation.

'Here's your ticket to Scotland,' the friendly receptionist told me. 'First class.'

I'd kept in touch with Frances by phone almost daily. She seemed pleased when I rang to say I was coming home, and by then I was certainly ready to be back with my family.

So, one more night in Denver. That evening Jack invited me to dinner in the hotel where we were both staying. We enjoyed drinks at the bar, but Jack had another surprise in store for me. After ordering our food in the restaurant, he immediately slumped into a deep sleep. There was nothing I could do! People were beginning to stare. I nudged him lightly. No response. I tried again. Still no movement from the burly Texan tycoon. There was not even a flicker from Jack; in fact, to make matters worse, he began to snore loudly.

As confused diners looked on I decided to eat my meal despite Jack's comatose state, brought on by sufficient quantities of a name to suit the occasion – Jack Daniels on the rocks.

My fellow diner woke up with a start, licked his lips, grunted, and gulped down a hearty measure of Jack Daniels from his tumbler. He attacked his gigantic T-bone steak as if nothing had happened while I looked on, more than a little embarrassed. I'd already finished my meal.

'Waitress, my steak is cold,' he grumbled loudly to the consternation of everyone inside the restaurant.

'What else could it be?' I murmured to myself as he complained bitterly. The 22-ounce specimen had lain on the plate for half an hour, unattended.

Jack seemed oblivious to the fact that he'd been asleep. He was barely aware of anyone else in the restaurant. All I could do was fill in the time and keep him quiet by talking while his fresh steak was being prepared. When another large section of cow arrived at the table, he devoured it with a vengeance.

After a while, with tears flowing down his face, he began opening up about personal problems he was having with his family. I assured him I would keep his confidence, and he replied that he knew that already.

The following day I left Denver, travelling via New York and London, and then on to Aberdeen. Back home Frances greeted me warmly, with no hint of the fury that had accompanied my departure.

In Aberdeen, I spent three or four nights a week at the dockside. I was fascinated by how the port was transformed into another world under darkness.

The energy of the place was really exciting, bustling with sailors, dockers, prostitutes, fishermen and oil workers. They filled the air with a variety of pungent aromas. All of the bars were full.

I regularly took our dog Arran with me and he'd play to the crowd, jumping up and putting his paws on my shoulders and generally revelling in all the attention that came his way.

I was beginning to earn good money with Hamilton

Brothers, and life in many ways was treating me well. Vicky and Louisa were no longer babies but little girls now, while our farmhouse had been converted into a lovely home. Frances drove a VW Scirocco, while I zoomed around in a Cortina XL estate. I had joined the Round Table in Stonehaven, south of Aberdeen, and we had a wide circle of good friends.

However, Frances was certainly not happy about my frenetic working environment. She still had a long-harboured dream of us buying and running a guesthouse on the Morecombe seafront; at twenty-three I was too much of a coward to tell her directly that this was never going to happen. I felt the time had come for me to start my own business.

I was starting to see extraordinary results from my four years of oil industry experience, and the overwhelming power of intention and desire. My years with Offshore Marine and Hamilton Brothers had served as a useful apprenticeship, but I aspired to work for myself and build my own business. And I knew that I was ready to start the journey.

My expertise was in stock control for Customs and Excise – keeping accurate company records covering the importing of oil well drilling equipment and other goods for oil exploration. I decided to use all of that experience to build my first business.

I registered a company called Exploration Production and Development LTD (EPD), and handed in my resignation at Hamilton Brothers. I'd befriended two other local businessmen, Malcolm Bradshaw and Brian Nimmo, who also worked for a company that served the oil industry, and we made plans to go into business together.

However, at the last minute they decided not to leave their employment and I was left on my own. Despite their decision, they still agreed to loan me £4,000 at 20% (in addition to a personal guarantee on our house) to start the business. When I saw my accountant he asked if he should register the new business for VAT. I thought this was not required, as the company was new and turnover wasn't likely to reach the necessary threshold in the foreseeable future. But within six weeks the company exceeded all expectations and I had to become registered. Caught up in a mood of optimism, I bought myself a white, second-hand MGB GT on hire purchase and a maroon MG Midget for Frances. I was on a roll.

My first stock control job was for a company in Montrose, a town an hour to the south of our house. I charged £3.50 an hour and was prepared to work whatever hours came my way. I put in sixty hours a week and that worked out at more than £200; a lot of money in those days. If a client asked for something I would make the effort to find and ship it. I remember moving welding rods in my MGB GT at night and then heading to Netherley, a short drive from our home near Stonehaven. A man called Bill Mennie manufactured pallets for me, and I sold them on for use in the oil industry.

I was starting to see real results from my efforts. I realised that I needed a proper base to deal with my expanding business. I took on more and more staff to deal with stock control as I launched new companies.

I had found my passion – being an entrepreneur. I believed that anyone, with enough determination and passion, could bring their dreams to life. Every barrier I challenged opened up even more opportunities, confirming film producer Samuel Goldwyn's quote, 'The harder I work, the luckier I get'.

I can only describe Aberdeen as Scotland's equivalent of The Goldrush. You had to be in Aberdeen in the Seventies to believe it. The city was buzzing and I gained the reputation of a problem solver. Oil and service companies were flooding the city with people and equipment.

By the age of twenty-four, I had several companies including the original stock control operation, now computerised, and a freight forwarding firm. Even then, I had seven years of experience in the oil industry.

My time had come. I was in the right place at the right time with the right people doing the right things. Day was the same as night; nothing stopped, and I was there to meet an insatiable demand. A twenty-four hour circus revolved around my life.

By then I could see other opportunities emerging. The whole area was booming and I found work a pleasure – and effortless.

I paid back the private loan of £4,000 within the first year of trading. At that point Malcolm Bradshaw, seeing my unexpected success, asked if he could become my business partner and we came to an agreement. He had a broad, ready smile and wore large aviator-style glasses.

We also both became Lloyd's underwriters, and then Malcolm, who had also worked as a session trumpeter, heard of a hotel and bar for sale next to the River Dee called The Mill Inn. We bought the premises, and converted the building into a nightclub and restaurant called Champers.

For our opening night we hired Legs and Co., the glamorous troupe from Top of the Pops who were the most famous dancers in the country at the time. It was a crazy, fun weekend. Champers was the first nightclub in Aberdeen and the best in Scotland. It had an enormous video screen and a hundred and forty four lights underneath a glass dance floor. It was copied from the set of Saturday Night Fever; in fact, the hits of Abba and the Bee Gees were anthems at Champers. Money, money, money poured in – and I hoped to win again! However, as Bachman Turner Overdrive told me in the Seventies, 'You Ain't Seen Nothin' Yet'.

We owned Champers for four years, entertaining the clubbers with disco music and top acts from the period. We even hosted the Miss Aberdeen contest on various occasions.

We always had an eye for a business deal. Malcolm and I entered the bidding for three minesweepers from the Royal Navy. These were Ham Class vessels, 120 feet long, with accommodation for thirty-five, and an 'A' frame on the rear to collect mines.

We were successful in acquiring one of them, HMS Downham, for £8,000! I could not believe the price. We took charge of the vessel in Portsmouth, but never actually went to see it. The port captain became so annoyed, after a few months, that he ordered us to attend to the vessel – or it would be impounded. The minesweeper required ropes manoeuvring with the tide. The furious port captain also demanded port dues. We advertised HMS Downham for sale. She was sold to a seismic company in the Med for £50,000; a handsome profit.

Peter Marshall, a friend who worked for an oil company, captured my imagination when he handed me a Sea Containers brochure. It gave details about conventional shipping containers used in the worldwide movement of goods. I was so busy that I didn't look at it for a while, but eventually I thumbed through; that moment became pivotal in my career.

Everything came flooding back. Memories of the Suffolk Shore, and losing all of that deck cargo in the storm, filled my head. At that moment I had a vision. I could see the cargo on the Suffolk Shore, tied to the deck on pallets. I could also see a brochure with steel containers, used to ferry cargo all around the world. But they weren't being used in the oil industry! I imagined the containers, properly lashed down on the Suffolk Shore instead of the hopeless palletised arrangement.

My motto: 'When something awful happens in your life, the seeds of something fantastic are also there. But, when this happens, will you recognise the opportunity? And, if you see that chance, will you do anything about it?'

I answered both of those questions that day by calling Sea Containers, found out all the prices, and hired one container immediately at the cost of eight shillings a day. I had the container sent to Aberdeen where steel slings were made to lift it. My investment for the year was only around £350, plus the cost of returning the container fully repaired at the end of the contract. My return on that container in one year was £1,500.

I was now in the container business, constantly reinvesting most of the profit into hiring more containers – and arranging contracts with customers. From hiring I moved into designing and buying. I could see the potential of this emerging market and took on a yard and workshop in the Tullos Industrial Estate in Aberdeen. Within two years, competitors had followed my lead – although I had over 80 per cent of the market and owned more than three thousand containers of all shapes and sizes.

I had been asked by Mobil Oil to supply thirty units of a specific sized container for a long-term rental, having agreed terms with one of their American employees, Calvin Seidensticker. He explained that he didn't have the paperwork completed, but asked me to proceed with their manufacture urgently. I was happy to do that and gave instruction for their build to start in Aberdeen.

Some weeks later, well into the manufacture of the container order, I was asked to go to Mobil's office to meet with their top man. I was invited into his plush office and sat down opposite Mr Obladaski, who looked like Danny DeVito, only far less attractive. He calmly told me that Mobil were cancelling their order, which was worth £20,000 to my company.

He then said that if I didn't accept this he would blacken my name and make sure that I never did business with Mobil again. I reminded him that Calvin had ordered the containers and I had accepted his word and that of Mobil's, and therefore I would not stop their manufacture. I added that if I halted their production I could not sustain the loss and it would ruin my business. He replied that he didn't care and repeated that he would ensure my name was mud if I pressed on. There was little point in continuing the conversation, so I declared that I would take Mobil to court and then left the room.

This was my first experience of litigation. I went to see my lawyer at Paull and Williamson, who also acted for Mobil. I was told that, since there was a conflict of interest, they would not be able to act for me, or Mobil. They directed me to another firm and I remember feeling pleasantly surprised that they had turned down acting for Mobil Oil.

A date was set for a court hearing some months ahead, shortly after a family holiday which I had already booked in Malta. While I was confident that I was in the right – especially as verbal contracts are considered binding under Scottish law – I nevertheless spent the entire holiday worrying about the possibility of losing. Me against Mobil Oil, y'all.

The day of the dreaded court case arrived, and Mobil's solicitor asked me on the court steps if I wanted to withdraw from the proceedings. I was confident that I had the evidence to support my case – and Calvin would be truthful when we called him as a witness. So I replied that I wanted to proceed. Hearing that, Mobil's solicitor walked over to his client.

The Mobil advocate, stern-faced, then walked over to me. Would they be pushing for something else, to ruin me completely? Were they going to really stick the knife in now? How could I take on a multi-billion dollar company?

Mobil's slick legal representative, normally used to high profile tussles against mighty corporations, told me: 'I have been instructed by my client to confirm with you that the case is being conceded.'

That was all he said. He didn't need to say anything else. And so, there on the court steps, at the very last moment, I had won my case against one of the world's largest corporations.

I had stuck to my guns and not succumbed to Obladaski's bullying. I felt like performing a Scottish reel on the steps of the court, but common sense got the better of me just in time.

I returned to my office to find a message asking me to

attend the office of Mobil Oil at noon that day. I arrived at their office, not far from my own building in Aberdeen, wondering if Obladaski would be there. He wasn't anywhere to be seen, and instead another American executive walked over to me and shook my hand. To my surprise, tea and biscuits were brought in. I waited for the elegantly dressed, thin and well-groomed American to make the first move.

'It's a pleasure to meet you, Mr Evans,' he beamed. 'May I call you Eric?'

'Please call me Eric,' I nodded.

'I have to tell you personally that I admire your fearless determination to proceed against all odds. There are few men who would ever have contemplated what you have done. This is not the way Mobil Oil should be dealing with suppliers.'

'I appreciate your honesty,' I admitted, wondering where this was leading.

'Just to clarify matters. The order for the containers still stands. I look forward to receiving them as soon as possible. In the future, all our container orders in Aberdeen will come from your company, EPD.'

I left the meeting in a jubilant mood and, true to the man's word, we received all of their business. Mr Obladaski was removed from his position in Mobil Oil.

I was ecstatic. My mission, as I had chosen to accept it, was a meeting in Aviemore, in the Highlands, the next day. As I drove along the valley floor with mountains on either side, my brand new Aston Martin Vantage was alone on the road. I replayed the events of the Mobil fiasco, with Climax Blues Band, pounding out of the radio, telling me 'Couldn't Get it Right'. Well I did get that one right.

I drove along, enthralled by the mountains, and appreciating the expensive roar of my Aston Martin. The cassette player boomed out Runrig's song about taking the high road and low road. I was in heaven.

At 7 a.m. on Christmas Day in 1977, I received a call from Shell Oil asking if I had three hundred and fifty mini containers. The caller explained that there had been a blow-out on one of their installations and they required the units urgently, to carry materials to plug the hole. I confirmed that I had three hundred and fifty containers, although I really only had forty available. On Christmas Day I had to borrow back my containers from companies who'd hired them – I sent out a fleet of trucks all over Aberdeen.

Obviously this was not the ideal day to tell my wife and children I was off to work, but that is how we built our success: by doing whatever was required for our clients at any time, day or night.

To make matters more complicated, it was a snowy day. However, I juggled the opening of presents with frantic calls to the office. I dashed home to play briefly with my daughters and grabbed a sandwich and a cup of tea, before returning to the docks.

As the day drew on and I had trucks heading in all directions, I managed to join my family for the quickest of Christmas dinners. By nightfall I had four vessels completely loaded, with two more to go. This was achieved just before midnight. The day was done, and so was I.

Some months later I was asked by Shell to quote for a two-year contract for a large quantity of containers of different sizes. After submitting the quotation I was invited to their offices to discuss the contract. I had a long wait outside and, when my turn eventually came, I could see twelve people sitting around a rectangular table in the boardroom. One man, chubby and greying, was obviously in charge of proceedings.

I was grilled intensely about my quotation and the price in particular – it was 20% higher than any of the other bids. I explained that we gave a comprehensive service using only our stock without hiring in, but was told that my prices were too high. I stood my ground, even though I had clearly offended a few people with my attitude and prepared to leave. I said that EPD would always be delighted to assist even if we did not win this contract.

The man at the head of the table, who had a quiet authority about him but had not yet spoken, asked: 'Are you the person I saw last Christmas down at the docks when we had a blow-out and needed three hundred and fifty containers urgently that day?'

'Yes,' I replied.

'I saw a white Range Rover throughout the day; were you co-ordinating the supply?'

'Yes,' I answered again.

'Why didn't you give the job to one of your people or share the day?' he asked.

'It was clearly an important job for you, requiring the best management; regardless that it was Christmas Day. That reflects the level of service EPD provides for its customers, especially as the job was so crucial for you.'

'The contract is yours!' he said, to the dismay of the Shell personnel around the table.

However, all the gains in professional terms were offset by definite losses to my private life. I was investing in all of my businesses, with trips to Egypt and Norway, and this took its toll on my relationship with my wife. The problems that had been evident in our marriage for quite some time were escalating.

On the surface we certainly had it all: in 1975 we had moved from the steading in Crawton to a beautiful, three-storey granite house in Queen's Road, in a smart part of Aberdeen. A year later we moved from there to Woodthorpe, a mansion in Bieldside, an exclusive suburb. Woodthorpe was a wonderful house, set along a tree-lined drive in eighteen acres with two cottages and a lake.

I had bought the house for £72,000 and then spent another £80,000 on renovating and furnishing the property, as well as adding a tennis court and garages for all the cars. To me, the property represented exactly what I had achieved. Not only did we have our dream house, but our daughters also attended Albyn, a top private school for girls. We also enjoyed family holidays to Malta, St Lucia, Barbados and Bermuda.

Frances and I also drove top-of-the range cars: my MGB GT had been traded in for a Jaguar XJS. In 1977, Jubilee Year, I bought a brand new silver Aston Martin Vantage and shortly afterwards a willow gold Rolls Royce Silver Shadow; meanwhile, Frances drove a Range Rover and a Mercedes 450 SL.

Cars have always been my passion, reflected in some of my other acquisitions at the time: a red E-Type Jaguar convertible, an original Mini Cooper and a completely renovated 1957 Aston Martin DB2/4 Coupe. On top of that we had two company planes, and for a while I took flying lessons.

I decided to learn to fly with Pegasus, the Aberdeen-based training club. My training took me one day to Inverness, in a Cessna 150. I had no idea that, after just ten hours at the controls, my trainer would suggest a solo flight. He thought I was ready.

Heartbeat up, legs shaking and with dampening hands, I prepared to perform the daring feat. As I taxied out to the threshold point, cleared for take-off, I proceeded down the runway. At this point my mind was 100% occupied with the flight! Nothing else entered my head. Talk about being on an island. I felt totally alone.

As I pulled back on the column I climbed quickly to 1,000 feet. I levelled off from a sky view to a horizon of land and sea, with mountains in the distance. I was petrified.

I completed my circuit – taking around half an hour – and prepared to land. I completely forgot the various tasks needed to land the aircraft. Would my ten hours of training really be enough to handle this?

I proceeded to my turning point to line up with the runway. Slowly and surely all of the instructions came flooding back. Sweat dripped from my hands. At 1,000 feet, the tower radio said: 'You are cleared to finals, number one'. For anyone who has flown solo, I know that you are with me here!

I heard the skid of the wheels as they touched the tarmac. What a relief. I proceeded down the runway and towards the parking area. Somehow, I'd made a perfect landing. The instructor told me that, although I was shaking like a leaf.

I shook like an even shakier leaf when I came in to land at Aberdeen, at that time Britain's second busiest airport. I was flying from the Dundee grass strip as part of my training – solo, of course.

Along the coast I flew, admiring the craggy coastline. It was late in the afternoon, and getting dark. I was cleared to land as number four, behind three other aircraft. However, I could only see two planes in front of me – not three.

'Abort,' the tower demanded. 'Continue on your circuit and we will confirm your landing position shortly.'

I was then cleared to land as number three, and this time I could see two other planes. The first one landed and, as I followed the next one, I was told to abort once more. This time the reason was the arrival of a BAC 1-11 behind me, and I was in the way. I was told to climb up to 1,000 feet and complete the circuit again. As I turned, I could see the jet landing beneath me.

Clouds enveloped my Cessna. I peered ahead through the darkness. I had no night training whatsoever, and so I was flying blind.

'I am a pilot learning to fly,' I stammered over the radio. 'I can't see the runway. I'm in cloud and it's dark. I can't see anything.'

Instant panic in the tower, with a message to all other traffic. 'A Cessna 150 is now cleared to land, number one.'

That meant that I was the top priority and the next to land.

'What can you see?' the controller in the tower asked me, with a fair degree of urgency.

'I can see intermittent street lights and houses.'

'Confirm when you are lined up with the runway,' the controller said, trying to sound calm.

As I turned to my downward leg, I could just see the runway lights though the clouds. As I slowly descended from five hundred feet I flew beneath the clouds and saw the runway clearly. I landed safely.

You can understand why I never flew solo again.

Apart from everything else going on, I sponsored a Royal Gala Variety Show in aid of the Prince's Trust at His Majesty's Theatre in Aberdeen, in October 1978.

On the night of the event Frances and I were introduced to Prince Charles, The Three Degrees and Michael Bentine of the Goons. I paid Michael's fee – worth every penny – and invited him for afternoon tea the following day. We spent a wonderful few hours together and he drew some cartoons that he signed and gave to Vicky and Louisa. He showed a real interest in our garden, in particular some rare rock formations, and produced a large carnelian crystal from his pocket.

'This is the stone of motivation, endurance, leadership and courage,' he enthused. 'Did you know that these stones have protected and inspired throughout history? I would like you to accept my personal stone as a gift.'

When Michael left, I read up more about carnelian stones. I learned that the crystal was iconic, dating back to Egyptian times. I still carry it in my pocket to this day.

Tom MacDonald, who looked after everything from the garden to my cars, ferried Michael and his wife around in the Rolls. Michael was interested in all sorts of monuments and stones; Tom enjoyed every moment, driving the celebrity all over the area to inspect the finest examples.

The following spring I received a letter of thanks from the Prince's Trust informing me that the Royal Gala Show had netted a final profit of almost £18,000, and I was so proud to have been a part of the event.

Regardless of all the superficial trappings in our life, Frances and I had grown so far apart that it seemed as if we had nothing in common except for our love for Vicky and Louisa. Our rows became even worse. Leaving the children was so difficult, but Frances and I could no longer live together. We parted late in 1978 and I went to live at Banchory Lodge, a beautiful Georgian hotel on the River Dee fifteen miles west of Aberdeen.

It was something of a haven for me, with the front lawn running down to the River Dee where salmon leapt in the waters. The owners, Dugald and Margaret Jaffray, were extremely welcoming and became an important part of my new life, although it was like living at Fawlty Towers. One morning as I was leaving for work I bumped into Dugald who was in abject panic, cursing and swearing because a guest had died overnight in the hotel.

'Selfish b*****d!' he exclaimed in his thick Scottish accent, his round face and blue eyes a picture of aggrievement. 'Who's going to pay that bill now?'

He wasn't joking – but I couldn't stop laughing at his genuine dismay at the inconvenience caused by the unfortunate death.

Dugald was on the short side, but what he lacked in height he certainly made up for with character. Later, when I returned from work, his description of getting the body removed from the hotel – while avoiding the other guests – was like a John Cleese sketch. There were lookouts on corridors, and guests unexpectedly appearing, with the body bag – finally, after three tortuous hours – being taken out to the waiting mortuary van via the kitchen. And, if laughter is the best medicine, then staying at Banchory Lodge was just what I needed at the time.

While my private life was definitely in turmoil, my business ventures were going from strength to strength. EPD had by then become the jewel in the crown of our business. From the solitary container that the company hired in the summer of '74, the business had mushroomed to owning three thousand, three hundred units, with 50% of the turnover being net profit. We quietly put it on the market and were approached by John Swire and Sons, a vast and well-respected conglomerate. Swire are based between London and Hong Kong and own Cathay Pacific. They spent a year doing due diligence checks on EPD and, finally satisfied, paid us £2 million for the company. The deal was finalised on my birthday – 2 March 1978.

'Dad,' I blurted out with excitement over the telephone. 'I've done it. The deal has gone through. I have a million in assets – now I also have it in cash. And I have the gold Rolls Royce and the number plate ESE 1.'

He said nothing. I remembered that day, aged seven, when he mocked my ambitions. I never understood why he ridiculed me then, and had nothing to say about my achievements twenty-one years later. I felt devastated and sad. I was back on my island.

I flew down to London in our new Piper Navajo Chieftain to join Malcolm who had gone on ahead. There were ten or so of us there to sign all the papers including solicitors, accountants, auditors and directors. It was a sensitive time as my heart and soul were very much in each individual container – unlike Malcolm, who had had limited involvement in running the business after becoming my partner.

I decided to put my father's indifference to the back of my mind. We celebrated with dinner at the White Elephant on the River in London that evening. Malcolm and I signed a three-year management contract with Swire, who had an insurance policy for £1 million on each of us. I was in a daze from it all. The following day we returned to Aberdeen with £2million in cheques. The bank manager said he had never had a deposit of such a large amount made in his career, and brought out a fine whisky from his cabinet.

As I felt the heat of the Scotch on my throat, I reflected on my rapid rise in the business world. We owned seven other companies around the world, including an early interest in the birth of wind power, computers and satellite communications. On one hand I felt I had really 'made it' in realising my dream; on the other, there was a gaping hole because I had sold my passion. Add to that the turmoil in my personal life with a divorce pending and uncertainly over arrangements with my children.

It should have been a wonderful time but, when reality kicked in, I felt a wave of unhappiness wash over me. I felt so lonely. I found out that money on its own didn't bring happiness.

I found out the hard way.

CHAPTER FOUR

In Search of Stalin's Gold

Kidney stone operation at St George's Hospital. Late June, 2014.

I'm woken the following morning at around 6.30 a.m. and change into a theatre gown and knee-length stockings to prevent blood clots. I'm continuing with a saline drip to keep hydrated, but otherwise it's been nil-by-mouth since late last night. The anaesthetist comes in to run through the process. The on-duty urologist says that he doesn't want stents inserted, but would rather the stones pass naturally. He is concerned that stents might cause blood loss or an infection and, with my compromised immune system and low platelet count, he would prefer to avoid that procedure if possible.

Through Anthony Nolan, Delete Blood Cancer UK and DKMS (the German equivalent), Axel has been informed that the procedure is on hold and he's sent me a text to find out how I am. He reassures me that, whenever I'm ready to go ahead again, he'll be ready as well. Once again I feel humbled by his attitude.

Early in the morning, the urologist informs me that they will not be inserting stents in my kidneys today, but will instead remove the stone in my left kidney with laser surgery after the weekend. From there the day continues with me being put back on a saline drip, receiving units of blood and platelets, plus Desferrioxamine injections. I also receive the Granulocyte-colony stimulating factor, (G-CSF) – a daily needle into my stomach to help stimulate my stem cell count.

The Desferrioxamine (or Desferal) is a binding agent that removes the excess iron from my constant transfusions, which my body cannot expel naturally. I've been taking this via a needle in the soft skin of my stomach from a slow-release pump for 12-14 hours a day, five days a week, since January. In addition I'm upping my water intake by mouth to try to pass the kidney stone naturally. Beyond that the day and evening follow the hospital routine, and I pass the time listening to music and watching the television.

The weekend passes quietly. I make calls to family or watch TV or catch up with emails, and the time is punctuated by a friend's visit in the afternoon. The anaesthetist describes the procedure for the operation on Monday. I am fortunate that the hospital has one of the country's leading kidney stone specialists, Mr Anson. Due to the medical complications of my case, he is the one performing the operation. Yet again, it feels as though luck is on my side.

Come Monday, I'm able to have breakfast at 6 a.m. and drink water until 2 p.m.; after that it's nil-by-mouth until my operation later on. I'm asked to walk down to have an X-ray to see if the stone has moved, but alas it is still in situ.

Back in my room I'm again given a theatre gown and knee stockings and asked to walk down to the theatre on the floor below, accompanied by the ward sister. Before long, Mr. Anson comes to see if I'm ready. I know I'm in good hands. I'm taken to the prep room where the anaesthetist is waiting.

She's soon inserting a cannula, connecting me to a heart monitor, asking whether I'm allergic to anything and about the antibiotics I'm receiving. Just before 5.30 p.m. the anaesthetic hits me and I'm asleep. As my eyes close, I recall another ocean-based adventure – this time an enormous money – spinner with a wartime theme.

★★★

When Frances and I separated late in 1978, I hoped that we could at least be civil with each other, but things between us were acrimonious from the start. By early the following year it was apparent that Frances and I would never be reconciled.

Her solicitor recommended that she should instigate divorce proceedings. All in all it was a bitter episode, with ugly accusations being flung in my direction.

Her solicitor used bogus claims to obtain a court order, restricting the time I could spend with Vicky and Louisa to a ridiculous three hours a week. My feelings were a jumble of anger and incredulity that Frances could be so cruel to her children. It was certainly a terrible phase for our daughters, caught as they were between us. Louisa later told me that, during all of this, she was unwavering in her love for me: I was her dad and, whatever happened, nothing would change between us. I was close to tears when she told me.

Some welcome respite: an eight-week business trip to Newfoundland in Canada. I'd sold a shipment of new containers to a start-up business in the oil industry. It was winter when I arrived in St John's, the capital of the province, which is built around a fairly small harbour sheltered in the shadow of a hill. The weather was brutal. Deep snow and frozen fog clung to the landscape and I was astonished to see the harbour blocked for days on end by a mountainous iceberg. A near neighbour, further out in the North Atlantic, sank the Titanic in 1912.

I had met this customer at the Oil Exhibition in Aberdeen. They were rapidly establishing themselves as suppliers to the offshore drilling industry in that part of Canada. This functioned in St John's, much the same as it did in Aberdeen – except for the additional constraints imposed by the icebergs. These are such a danger because an iceberg travelling at just a few miles an hour can sink most structures in its path. As a result, companies have put 'Ice Management Programs' in place to monitor icebergs and, if required, send support vessels to tow them away. Only around a tenth of an iceberg lies above the surface; they can weigh 200,000 tons.

My hotel was close to the harbour and, on most days, I was collected in a large truck with snow chains and taken to various warehouses and offices. At the time, St. John's was predominantly a fishing port. The harbour was always an interesting place with all manner of vessels coming and going – when not locked in ice – and I spent many a pleasant hour in a harbour-side cafe taking everything in. I was shocked to see flipper pie on the menu, a traditional local dish cut from young harp seals, and also fishermen selling flippers for 50 cents each. In the evenings I usually stayed in to eat at the hotel, as the sidewalks were impassable with snow and it was far too cold to venture outside.

By the time my work was finished I was happy to leave and get back to see Vicky and Louisa – even if Frances remained as difficult as ever about me seeing them – and also my work routine in Aberdeen. Dealing with my divorce was more arduous, but thankfully by the spring of 1980 it was all over.

By then I was living in a cottage on the Lower Deeside Road, a few miles upriver from Champers towards Aberdeen, with Chester, Babushka and Aston – three Persian cats I bought for the children.

Despite a lot of attention from women at the nightclub, it was mostly a difficult period. Within a short time I'd sold my company, divorced, and hardly got to see my daughters. To try to redress this I bought the girls a horse each as they were both keen and accomplished riders, competing in showjumping and cross-country events. Louisa's horse stood 12.2 hands and was a beautiful Welsh part Arab dapple grey mare called Rosland Blue Bonnet. Vicky's horse, Fairholme Dianthus, stood at 13.5 hands; they also shared a pony called Smokey Joe.

I stabled all the horses at a farm owned by my friend Sheila, so that the girls and I could spend more time together beyond the draconian restrictions of the court order. Sheila, a striking blonde lady, six feet tall, strode around the stable yard in wellington boots and a long fur coat. She made us feel most welcome. The farm became a tranquil haven where the girls and I spent many a happy hour, apart from a day when Sheila's goat ate my Aston Martin's aerial! It was the fastest car in production at the time, travelling from 0-60mph in 5.2 seconds – with or without the aerial.

When the divorce was finalised, I threw some money at soothing my pain. I splashed out on an Aston Martin Volante convertible in Windsor red and booked a holiday on my own to Fort Lauderdale in Florida. I stayed at the Hilton Hotel on Galt Ocean Mile and forced myself out of my comfort zone by making the effort to talk to everyone. It was time to finally have some fun after the stress and strain of the past few years.

One night I was drinking vodka in the bar and listening to a group playing background music.

'*I met her in a club down in old Soho. Where you drink champagne and it tastes just like cherry cola.*'

Eh? I sipped the vodka, a little worse for wear, thinking: 'I know that tune and I recognise that voice.'

I peered through the smoky haze to see Ray and Dave Davies and the rest of the band performing. I could scarcely believe it. The Kinks were playing live!

I made so many friends in Florida that I later went on holiday with them to Bermuda, Las Vegas and New York.

I returned from New York on Concorde. What an experience, even in a confined space.

'BOOM.'

The graceful supersonic aircraft broke the sound barrier when we headed out over the Atlantic at 670 mph.

'Mach 2,' the pilot announced as we streaked through the sky at twice the speed of sound, 1,340 mph, at a height of eleven miles. A sudden surge of power pushed me back in my seat.

I felt as though I was travelling through time and space, at twenty-three miles a minute. A fellow passenger told me that the aircraft expanded up to ten inches due to the friction and heat generated. The wingspan is only eighty four feet, so every little helps.

Three hours and forty five minutes after take-off, and my bank balance £875 lighter for the one-way trip, I arrived in London. I chatted to a passenger who had flown to America to buy a book the same day. Bizarre.

I stepped off Concorde and into the more humble surroundings of a BAC 1-11, which had no chance of threatening the sound barrier. The aircraft ploughed on to Aberdeen; and I flew ever so slowly and noisily back to reality.

Back in Aberdeen Malcolm and I were approached by Ric Wharton, a deep-sea diver who was looking to fund a unique adventure. Ric and his partner, Malcolm Williams, ran a highly successful diving company, Wharton Williams, and they had been invited to join a salvage operation on HMS Edinburgh.

On 2 May, 1942, HMS Edinburgh was bombarded relentlessly during a running battle with German destroyers and a U-boat. Sixty of the Royal Navy warship's crew were killed.

Minutes after her remaining crew were saved, she was sunk by a torpedo fired from a destroyer in the Edinburgh's convoy, with the dead men still on board. The cargo had to be kept secret.

The project was spearheaded by Keith Jessop, an ex-Royal Marine who had won the rights to dive on the wreck of the Edinburgh. She lay more than eight hundred feet down in the icy waters of the Barents Sea in the Arctic Ocean. At the time, this was the deepest salvage ever attempted, and Keith had spent years investigating and planning the project.

What made this salvage operation of particular interest

was the top-secret consignment that the cruiser had been carrying when she went down – vast amounts of gold bullion. The Edinburgh was on the homeward journey from the Soviet Union, where she had escorted seventeen merchant ships from the west coast of Scotland that had just delivered tanks, planes and other vital war supplies. Russia's payment for these munitions, which the Edinburgh carried, was four hundred and sixty five gold bars – five tonnes of gold – packed in ninety-three rough wooden boxes. On board: Stalin's Gold, bearing the stamp of an eagle.

By the time the consortium of treasure hunters approached us, they had already found the wreck and sent down a robot camera. HMS Edinburgh had been designated a war grave in 1957, which meant that no explosives could be used to retrieve the gold. As a result a team of the best deep sea divers from around the world – who also had the necessary skills to cut through the armour-plating on the Edinburgh's hull – had been assembled. The most technically advanced diving vessel of the time, the Stephaniturm, complete with a three-man diving bell, was lined up for the operation.

All that the project lacked now was the funding to proceed. Even though most of the individuals and even companies involved were working on a 'no find, no fee' basis, there were still many other expenses involved. Malcolm and I were offered a return of six to one on our investment, and we were more than happy to put in £25,000 cash each.

We were prepared to wait and see what happened, with the salvage operation planned for a few weeks' time.

Meanwhile, I continued with the running of EPD. Amongst other things, I was organising a stand at an Oil Exhibition in Aberdeen. We planned to entertain clients during the week of the show, with events at Champers every night and also in the hot-air balloon we co-owned with Pegasus Flying Club.

Our stand looked like a film set. They were always designed

to grab attention and this year was no different, working with an ancient Roman theme. The all-white set, complete with Roman pillars, was made even more attractive by the presence of Miss Edinburgh, Miss Glasgow, plus two other attractive friends of mine, Wendy and Janice. They looked like the cast of Charlie's Angels. A friend, Darlene Cox, had designed their costumes. They were eye-catching, to say the least, consisting of gold-trimmed white mini togas and towering gold high heels.

On the first morning of the exhibition I had arranged for the four women to be in their costumes, ready for collection at Darlene's dress shop. I was in my willow gold Rolls with the number plate ESE1, and we drew some curious glances as we set off towards the exhibition centre.

Unfortunately we hit a traffic queue when we reached the dual carriageway. The queue stretched for miles, even though it was only 7.30 a.m. and I was worried that we'd be late. Then a police bike pulled up alongside the car. I was shocked, wondering what traffic offence I might have committed.

I needn't have worried. I had healthy relationships with the police, including this particular officer who happened to be a good friend. He beckoned me out of the queue and into the clear lane, while stopping the rest of the traffic from doing the same. He put on his blue flashing light and escorted us at speed all the way past the stationary drivers – who were looking at us in amazement – to the exhibition centre. We certainly made quite an entrance amongst the gathering crowds. After I came to a halt I thanked my friend, and he just smiled back and sped off. And if I hadn't attracted the women's attention before that, well…

The week was rounded off nicely when Malcolm and I received a call from Rick Wharton that a diver on the salvage operation on HMS Edinburgh had retrieved the first bar of Stalin's Gold. It had been expected that the gold bars, which on average weighed 11.9 kilos each, would have the stamp of the Tsarist eagle; in fact, all had Soviet markings. Over the next few weeks, until bad weather swept in and halted the dive until the following year, four hundred and thirty one gold bars were extracted from the wreck – worth roughly £45 million at the time – and the project was described by The Sunday Times as 'quite simply, the greatest salvage operation in the annals of the sea'. A total of £9 million went to the Soviet government,[4] while the British government took £4.5 million, and the rest was divided proportionately amongst the project consortium.

The salvage also broke all previous records for deep sea diving, as divers remained under the sea in compression chambers for forty-two days. Nobody had worked at that depth and in that cold before. I was offered the choice of whether to take a gold bar or cash, and perhaps unwisely chose money. The gold bar was worth around $100,000 – and rising.

A few months later, as my contract with Swire approached its end, I was still seeing very little of Vicky and Louisa, while my relationship with their mother remained volatile, to say the least. I just didn't seem to be able to find any peace with my situation. I started to think more and more about making a fresh start away from Aberdeen and, after a great deal of consideration, decided that the tax haven Jersey – being close enough to my daughters but far enough from my ex-wife – would make an ideal place for me to call home.

While it was easy for me to tell Frances about my decision, it was the most difficult conversation to have with Vicky and Louisa. It took them a while to get used to the idea. Stepping down from work was probably the easiest part to deal with, as by then my contract with EPD had ended and I knew that I was

4   The Russians had shown exactly how interested they were in the bullion by anchoring two vessels within a short distance of the *Stephaniturm*. They also had representatives on board the dive ship to monitor the whole salvage operation.

leaving the company in excellent shape. I sold the cottage I'd bought after staying in Banchory Lodge, as well as its contents, and had my Aston Martin Volante taken to Jersey along with a few boxes of personal effects.

On the morning of my departure, all that I had to do was pack my bedding and a few other small items into my Rolls Royce. I said a final goodbye to a loyal friend in a pub near Aberdeen. It was a sunny day early in April 1982, and I had mixed emotions as I drove away from the city, and then past Champers Nightclub, which I still co-owned. Eventually I reached the top of a hill where I stopped and looked back at the now distant views of Aberdeen. I was feeling increasingly lonely and sad, especially about leaving behind my children. However, apart from them, little else remained of my former world there. I forced my thoughts towards my new life on the island of Jersey.

Suddenly, I realised that the faster I could put distance between me and Aberdeen the better, and I drove at some speed past Stonehaven, then Perth, Glasgow, and on through the Lake District, past Manchester, Birmingham and finally towards Southampton. I arrived in Hampshire feeling mentally and physically shattered. It had been the most difficult of days, but my mind was more focused on where I was going than where I'd been.

I spent that night in Southampton before boarding the ferry to the Channel Islands. There was no sight of land when I woke for breakfast the following morning, but shortly afterwards Jersey appeared on the horizon. Before long, as we passed Corbiere lighthouse and came around the coast to St Brelade's Bay, the sun was shining and flooding the ferry's lounge. For the first time in days I felt warm and comfortable. It was high tide as we came into St Helier. After docking we disembarked and I drove the short distance to the Grand Hotel – my home for the foreseeable future.

As I locked the car door and looked out across the bay I realised that, only thirty-six hours earlier, I had left Aberdeen; somehow it seemed a lot longer than that.

I remembered the friendly receptionist who had been exceptionally helpful when I made my reservation, making sure that I had a double room with a desk for an indefinite time. Her name was Sue Werry and she had made a great impression on me during that conversation. I was now keen to meet her.

I didn't have long to wait. Sue was a feast for my travel-weary eyes. I remembered her attractive voice from our phone conversation; her long blonde hair glinted as the sun streamed into the reception area; she had thoughtful, intelligent blue eyes; her clothes were immaculate. I was bowled over. Sue showed me to my room and wished me a pleasant stay. I asked her to find me quickly if my daughters rang.

After unpacking, I strolled across to the beach where I sat down in a cafe to take in the atmosphere and enjoy the spring weather. I literally had no plans other than to enjoy the sunshine and learn to ride a horse, something I had promised myself for Vicky and Louisa.

My only other riding experience had been during a family holiday in St Lucia. The guide turned up with a string of animals that he allocated according to how each rider declared their ability. Having handed out horses to the other five members of the group, our guide then gave me my animal, which admittedly had four legs, a tail and sported a saddle. However, it was a donkey.

Neither the donkey nor I had a good time that day. The donkey alternated between refusing to budge and then accelerating without warning into an out-of-control canter that had me bouncing in and out of the ill-fitting saddle like a jumping jack. It clearly did not want me on its back – emphasising this point by biting me so hard on the leg that I was left with deep teeth marks in my skin.

The whole experience had put me off riding but, for the sake of my daughters who loved the sport, I was willing to make the effort to learn properly. Most mornings I went to the Wagon Wheel cafe near the Grand Hotel for a bacon sandwich and tea before heading for a riding lesson in St Peter's Valley. The stable owner was incredibly patient in teaching someone whose natural talent for the sport proved to be negligible.

Thankfully most lessons ended in laughter and not tears and then a much needed cup of tea with my teacher, before driving down to St Brelade's Bay – the best beach on the island. And that became my ritual on Jersey for several months as I slowly got to know the island in general and the people at the hotel. Many of the staff also frequented the Wagon Wheel, including Sue, the bookings supremo, and we gradually became friends. She was twenty, from Cumbria, and beautiful in every way.

Gradually my riding improved, and by the time Vicky and Louisa came over for their first visit to the island I was thrilled at the prospect of surprising them. I took them to the stable in St Peter's Valley where another Sue, my riding instructor, helped to choose our horses.

We enjoyed a canter along the quiet country road and all seemed to be going well. Out of the blue my horse bolted and we were galloping along; however, I was completely out of control. The horse's head was down, its ears back, and it felt like we were travelling at seventy miles an hour. I was bouncing all over the place and just managed to stay on the horse. I pulled on the reins and sat deep in my saddle, but this made no difference.

By then I'd lost sight of Vicky and Louisa, but thankfully Sue soon caught up alongside. Somehow, she managed to take the reins and bring the sweating, frothing animal to a halt. When we returned to the stable I was relieved that I hadn't seriously injured myself. As I dismounted, I vowed never to go riding again

– adding to my self-imposed restrictions on boats and aircraft.

I was slowly learning to have a life other than that of work and to seize the moment and have fun. One day, on a whim, I packed a bag, drew out £5,000 from the bank, jumped in my Aston Martin convertible and onto the ferry to St Malo. From there I drove the twelve hundred miles down to Marbella, enjoying the wind in my hair and the sun on my face. The downside to this hedonism hit me right between the eyes; literally. I was knocked out for three days by sunstroke and a blinding headache. But lesson learned – to wear a hat when it's sunny and the roof is down on a convertible car!

Three friends of mine arrived from Aberdeen and the next three weeks passed in a blur, trawling the bars of Puerto Banus, a marina to the southwest of Marbella.

One morning in the early hours, I was returning from Sinatra's Bar in the marina when two long-legged, mini-skirted girls put their thumbs up for a lift. Of course I stopped to pick them up.

'Life doesn't get better than this,' I thought as, without a word, the 'girl' beside me gently put her hand on my knee.

'How are you doing?' she asked, not in a feminine way, but in a deep, gravelly man's voice.

Clearly, I had unwittingly picked up two transvestites! I took the guy's hand off my knee and turned to look at him and his friend.

'Why don't we go to James Hunt's nightclub and have a good time with this situation?' I suggested.

They both seemed happy with the idea and so we drove to the club. We drew up at the front of the venue where, despite the hour, there was still a line of people at the door.

'Join the queue while I park the car and I'll see you at the bar,' I said, handing one of them a suitable amount of cash.

'I'll have a pint,' I added, before putting my foot on the accelerator and high-tailing it away.

Back in Jersey I began spending more and more time with Sue the receptionist, and before long we were very much an item and becoming increasingly close. Vicky and Louisa came over to Jersey to stay with me at The Grand, and they, too, loved Sue. I saw more of the girls in Jersey than I did in Aberdeen. Life was really improving for me.

Nevertheless, I was certainly not ready to spend every day playing golf and I really missed the buzz of a business deal. Malcolm and I still had Champers and other interests in the States and Canada. I decided to head to Lafayette in Texas where we had invested in a ground-breaking business, manufacturing precision down-hole tools for the oil industry using computerised lathes. From there, I went on to Halifax, Nova Scotia, where there was talk of drilling starting off-shore.

Even though I was only thirty-one, by then I had been in the oil business for fourteen years and knew a great deal about onshore supply bases and operations. Halifax Harbour is a large natural inlet on the Atlantic side of Nova Scotia.

At the time there was an established port area on the Halifax side that attracted all the local business, totally controlled by the dockers' union. On the other side of the water is less-developed Dartmouth. There, I found a scrapyard that had edged its way into existence beside the water; I managed to negotiate an option to buy the site over a two-year period. If the planned offshore drilling was successful, then we would have a bonanza with the five-acre site not controlled by the dockers.

The project took me to Halifax for stretches of a month or so several times over the next few years. I was fascinated to learn about Sable Island,[5] a thin ribbon of land twenty-six miles

---

5   On December 1st 2013 Sable Island was granted full status as a Canadian National Park Reserve and its fragile ecology is now for evermore protected by law.

long but only half a mile wide, set precariously and all alone at the edge of the continental shelf in the Atlantic Ocean – some two hundred miles southeast of Nova Scotia. Because of its location, the island is often in the path of strong hurricanes and also frequently engulfed by thick fogs; together these have caused three hundred and fifty recorded ships to fall victim to its sandbars.

The island has hundreds of species of birds either in permanent residence or in migration, as well as being a breeding ground to vast numbers of harbour and grey seals. It is also home to the iconic Sable Island ponies, which are believed to have been first introduced to the island in the 18th century to assist in the rescues after a shipwreck. They are an exceptionally hardy breed that roam freely and number around five hundred, only growing to about fifty-four inches tall due their diet of marram, the tough island grass.

Halifax was also the scene of a disaster that killed two thousand people and injured another nine thousand. In the First World War, the Royal Navy kept the Atlantic sea lanes open by using Halifax as its North American base. On the morning of December 6, 1917. SS Mont-Blanc, a French cargo ship fully loaded with wartime explosives, was involved in a collision with the Norwegian vessel SS Imo in the Narrows. This strait connects the upper Halifax Harbour to Bedford Basin. A fire on board the French ship ignited her explosive cargo, causing a cataclysmic explosion that devastated the Richmond District of Halifax. It was the most devastating man-made explosion in the pre-atomic age.

While summers in Halifax were great – and it was an interesting city with a rich history, much of which reflected the evolution of North America – winter was awful. One evening I left the office on the Dartmouth side to catch the ferry to downtown Halifax. It was –32 degrees Celsius with a vicious wind. It felt as though it could not get any colder. I was wrapped suitably apart from my face and ears and anxious not to fall in the deep snow. I made it easily to the harbour and was inside during the short ferry ride, but when I disembarked it was hard to breathe; the air was that cold.

As I walked along the quayside I realised that I wouldn't make it back to my hotel in one go, and decided to split my journey by visiting a restaurant along the way. As I opened the door the heat from the open fire hit me and I was given an equally warm welcome by the Glasgow family who ran it.

I sat by the fire and ate an Aberdeen Angus steak, accompanied by a wonderful red Bordeaux, before continuing the last half mile up the hill. By the time I reached my hotel I was frozen and shaking, and my ears felt as if they would shatter into pieces if I touched them. I found that a couple of large brandies were a satisfactory remedy. Subsequently, I either left Dartmouth earlier, or took a taxi from the ferry to the hotel. However, after an extended period of high investment we decided to close our endeavours in Halifax as there were no significant oil or gas finds during that time; nonetheless, it had been an exciting experience.

Returning to Jersey after each of my trips to Canada only highlighted the growing bond between Sue and me. During my first summer with Sue she invited me join her on holiday with her parents at their apartment in Spain. I had arranged to meet up with friends in Monaco and said that I would drive from there to meet her and her parents off the plane in Malaga. I took the Aston down through France and stayed in the Monte Carlo Grand Hotel – now called the Fairmont – which forms the tunnel of the Grand Prix circuit. After five days I set off to enjoy the drive down to the south of Spain. Naively, I hadn't given much thought to the drive from Monaco to Malaga, and imagined that two days of driving would suffice for the eight hundred mile trip.

The first day driving along the coastal road in France was

time consuming enough, as the road meandered much more than I'd anticipated, but I was in shock as I crossed the border into Spain during that summer of '82. The roads were at best poor and terribly maintained. For long stretches there weren't even roads near the coast, adding many more miles to the journey. There were also great distances when I had to drive at a walking speed to prevent damaging the car. At other times I was forced to a halt by new motorway construction, which enveloped the Aston in choking dust. Thankfully, the car had air conditioning.

I was becoming increasingly anxious about not reaching the airport in time to meet Sue off her flight at 5 p.m. the next day. Finally, exhausted, I checked into a hotel at 1 a.m, collapsed into a deep sleep and booked out only six hours later. I made it to Malaga Airport ten minutes before her flight arrived, though I was pretty dishevelled from exhaustion and my beautiful metallic deep-red Aston was covered in sand-coloured dust.

Her parents, Gordon and Jean, were most welcoming, and we had a fantastic few days together, laughing and telling stories. At the end of our holiday there, Sue and I had agreed to drive slowly north up through Spain and France and back to St Malo for the ferry to Jersey.

On our last night in France, we realised that, if we raced a little, we could catch an earlier ferry. The next morning we pushed on, with Sue – who was facing the traffic on the left hand side in my right hand car – telling me whether the road was clear for me to overtake. Sue became adept at judging the traffic and we ate up the miles. Just south of Rennes, about an hour and a half from St Malo, this (in hindsight very foolish) game was brought to an abrupt stop by the blue flashing light and siren of a police car.

I had arrogantly become used to driving the Aston at high speeds on French motorways, so in my mind driving at

100mph didn't really seem that fast to me. Unfortunately, the French police didn't see eye to eye with me on that matter.

We were pulled off the main road into a side street just outside a village. I was told to get out of the car and into a large van where three gendarmes were all clamouring to show me my speed on camera.

Ooops. It was difficult to deny but easy to say that I didn't speak French, and fortunately none of them spoke English. Nonetheless, this was serious and I knew it. For over an hour Sue sat demurely in the car while the policemen continued their circular non-conversation with me and occasionally tried to charm Sue, who they obviously thought was most attractive.

Eventually another police car drew up with four capped officers inside. I was now really worried. The new police officers tried out their best pigeon English on me while I continued to act dumb. They were clearly unsure of what to do with the Jersey registered car and its two occupants with whom they couldn't communicate. For a while they simply stared at the car and then one of them, using hand signals, asked me to lift the bonnet and they all looked approvingly at the V8 5.4 litre engine.

Then three of the new officers approached me and I imagined a spell in prison. But, no, their arrival had signalled a change in shift, and the officers who had stopped me didn't want to hang around on a Saturday night to sort out the paperwork on a speeding foreign car.

While the first batch of policemen drove away, I was given a thorough telling off and then beckoned to leave. I started the car and slowly pulled away with a shy wave, thanking my lucky stars while Sue roared with laughter. We drove reasonably slowly and still made the ferry back to Jersey.

Later that year, in November, the Jersey government approved my residency, finally allowing me to buy property and live on the island. It had taken so long because the local government carried out thorough checks on all applicants. I was the poorest of the ten new residents who were allowed in that year! The Grand Hotel had, by then, been my home for eight months. The prestigious building on the seafront had been a marvellous place to stay, but I was ready to have a home of my own again.

I found a three-bedroom, two-bathroom apartment with a wrap-around balcony near the top of a block overlooking the harbour and Elizabeth Castle in St Helier. I knew that Vicky and Louisa would love the place.

Early in 1983 I began investing in Benetton, the Italian clothing franchise, having been introduced to the brand by an old friend in Aberdeen. I opened the first shop there in Union Street, followed shortly afterwards by shops in Inverness, Stirling and Ayr. In just over a year I had fourteen Benetton shops throughout Great Britain from Aberdeen to the Isle of Wight. I was enthusiastic to start with, but as the amount of work piled up I began to lose interest.

The margins were low, and so I sold some of the shops and closed others. In the end, I found that I had made more profit trading property than multi-coloured pullovers. Benetton and I parted company. I left Benetton in my rear view mirror, several years before their appearance in Formula One and astonishing success with Michael Schumacher.

Little did I know, as this chapter of my life closed, that my future travel plans were almost a formula for disaster.

CHAPTER FIVE

Terror at Orly

Kidney stone treatment continues at St George's Hospital.

I 'come to' in the recovery room and beside me a woman is filling in a great deal of paperwork. I'm very groggy, but by 7 p.m. I'm feeling considerably better. I ask about my kidney, which feels sore, and I'm told that the stone was crushed by the laser, so no stent or catheter was required.

As I slowly wake up I reflect on how brilliant the NHS is. I am so grateful to the Ruth Myles Day Unit where I receive weekly blood transfusions, the Isolation Unit and also the Renal Unit. I am so impressed with all the staff and their unstinting dedication.

Soon, I'm taken by trolley back to my room where I have a light meal and call and text my family. I fall asleep, reflecting on how well the day has gone.

The following morning I'm up and dressed by 7.30 a.m. Pain has kept me awake for much of the night as there was a mix-up with the nurse who told me I'd had my allowance of painkillers. I spent many of those hours reflecting on how precious life is and the importance of making every moment count in some way.

I eat breakfast and Mr Anson's assistant comes by to see how I am. He's followed a while later by the oncology team who will monitor me for another 24 hours and then I'll probably be allowed home. The rest of the day passes uneventfully, with regular checks by the many staff monitoring my health. I ask for and receive sleeping pills and get a better night's sleep.

The following morning the two oncologists overseeing my case, as well as Mr Anson who operated on my kidney stone, all visit me. They're pleased with my progress and I'll be discharged later today, returning in two days to have my blood checked. Next Monday I am due to resume my regular weekly visits to have blood and platelet transfusions until my bone marrow transplant can be rescheduled, which will probably be in four to six weeks.

I wait to receive a final bag of platelets before being discharged, as well as additional medication to take home from the hospital pharmacy (Aciclovir, Tamsulosin, Lenograstim, Itraconazole, Zopiclone and Quinine Sulphate). I use the time to reflect on the ups and downs of life that can rise and then fall as sharply as the line on the cardiac monitor. Right now I have three main priorities in life: regaining my health; enjoying my family and friends; and reclaiming some freedom – by which I mean the ability to make choices.

I've had a tough few years, with a court case in which I was a witness for the prosecution, the decline in my health, and the total collapse of my finances. But then I've been there before – at least with the last two on that list.

As I wait to be discharged, I close my eyes and re-live an atrocity which will haunt me for the rest of my life. It is a vivid image, probably caused by the morphine, and I am transported back to a horrific incident more than thirty years ago. My resting heartbeat is 62 beats per minute. The four-hourly checks reveal that my drug-induced nightmare pushed that figure up to 90. My body is responding to an awful memory.

★★★

Early on 15 July 1983, I caught the morning flight from Jersey to Charles De Gaulle Airport in Paris. It was the height of summer: hot, with a perfect deep blue sky. The flight was uneventful and I landed, collected my luggage, taking the transfer bus to Orly Airport for a connecting flight down to Malaga. I'd never been to Orly Airport before, so it was a new experience. On arrival I picked up my bags and joined the other passengers in the elegant, glass-fronted terminal.

Once inside, I looked slowly around to get my bearings and find the check-in for the flight to Spain. The airport didn't appear busy and, in keeping with the summer holiday season, there was a relaxed atmosphere. I took my time, unaware that these few seconds would soon become the difference between life and death.

It seemed that passengers could check in for any flight from any queue, so I joined the shortest line, and was about fifth or sixth in the row. At the front stood a family of four; I distinctly remember because the children, a boy and a girl of about four and five, were so excited. Behind them were all individual travellers, and then me. The line moved rapidly when the family left the desk. The dark-haired, French woman at the check-in was quick and efficient and all smiles.

Behind me was a man I remember more for his battered bag than anything else. He was dressed in dark, anonymous clothes and looked unassuming. I just glanced at him and then my gaze swept along the queue forming behind. I noticed several faces from my bus journey.

I handed my ticket to the woman at the counter, as I had done hundreds of times in endless airports around the world. She quickly checked me in and my bag disappeared out of sight on the conveyor belt. As I turned to my left to walk away the man behind me lifted his case to take the place of mine. Within seconds I had stepped behind a wide pillar that supported the roof of the impressive terminal. The terminal had filled up with people and I didn't want to be in the way of the general flow. I knelt down to open my briefcase and put in my papers before going through customs.

Boom! Bang! A burst of light stunned my eyes. I couldn't breathe. I had never seen such a bright light; I had never heard such a loud noise. As I stumbled around in the confusion, an eerie silence settled over the hall. A rush of air gave way to the sound of shattering glass, making another terrifying noise. My ears were numb; my brain was in a daze; my senses were transported to a different place. The normal hubbub of the airport terminal was replaced by a ghastly scene from a horror movie, all happening before my eyes in vivid colour and in agonising slow motion.

Within moments I was surrounded by the shards of glass of all shapes and sizes while the hall also filled with the desperate screams of mothers and children, all naturally terror-stricken. The pillar had most certainly saved my life, as there were piles of glass to the left and right of me. Miraculously, I had been spared.

The air was full of smoke; the horrid tang in my nostrils reminded me of bonfire night. I was enveloped in an odd, swirling mist, which appeared around me almost as if in slow motion. The mist and its contents crashed continuously against the lifesaving pillar. I felt as if I was choking.

Three metres from me I could see a young woman, brunette, probably in her mid-thirties. She was covered in blood and repeatedly screaming her child's name in French. The panic in her face will haunt me forever. After those screams, all I could hear, in various languages, was: 'It's a bomb. It's a bomb.'

Eight people were killed that day and more than fifty injured. It transpired that the man behind me in the queue was a terrorist trying to check in a suitcase to blow up the plane. The Semtex had exploded too soon.

The bomb, planted by the militant group ASALA, had gone off at the check-in desk. ASALA threatened French interests around the world, as they claimed the Armenian people were being victimised.

I stood up, holding my case, to find the hall in chaos. With the front of the terminal blown out, people were pouring from the building in absolute panic. Bodies lay still beside the check-in desk, bloodied and clearly dead, and the walking wounded staggered around dazed or sat stunned with blood-covered faces and clothing. I was also very conscious of the possibility of another explosion and cautious about where I went. My thoughts turned to Vicky and Louisa, who I presumed were safe at home, and I felt so grateful that they had not been with me. At that moment, all I wanted to hear was their voices.

Soon a multitude of sirens added to the chaos and confusion; the frantic screams of mothers for their lost or injured – or, God forbid – dead children. I was in shock and struggling to keep up with the events unfolding in front of me.

At some point a calm voice came over the loudspeaker. The male voice, alternating between French and English, announced that the airport was closed. He asked everyone to evacuate the building and to wait on the road opposite the entrance for further instructions. I walked past the pillar that saved my life. It was the only area without broken glass.

Hundreds of people congregated outside the entrance where legions of ambulances were lined up. Medics streamed inside to attend to the injured. Glass crunched beneath my feet as I stumbled through the building. I was still in a state of shock. Blood was splattered everywhere. A musky smell hung in the air, along with a thick dust. The summer sun was blotted out. The terminal felt like a war zone.

As I walked to join the throngs outside, there was a clear separation between those who had survived unhurt, and those who had not. Looking back towards the building, the airport frontage was now gone; in its place was a tangle of steel and cables, peaks of jagged glass, and frantic people trying to administer first aid. A tangle of wires resembled strands of spaghetti blowing in the wind.

We stood mostly silent in the July midday sun – the shrill of sirens too loud to talk over – realising how lucky we were to have survived the blast. What if I'd stayed a moment longer in front of the pillar? What if I'd lingered for another second or two, close to the terrorist? I certainly wouldn't be here today, writing this.

Before long the press arrived: TV crews, reporters and photographers swarmed around the airport. Some of the survivors started taking photos, hoping to sell them, and reporters came over asking for eyewitness accounts. I was still deafened by the explosion. I just kept quiet and moved as far away as the police would allow, out of sight and sound of people who wanted to profit from such misery.

Three hours later the airport reopened; ironically, my original boarding pass and completed paperwork were still intact, ready for my next attempt to get onto an aircraft.

The bombing changed me. I lost some innocence that day and realised how fragile life is and how often fate rests in others' hands. Possibly for the first time in my life I felt truly vulnerable and prayed that I would never be in a situation like that again. Little did I know that events in Liberia would, one day, do just that.

Around this time, I was introduced to an engineering company based near Glasgow. They manufactured and renewed drill pipe for the oil and gas industry, mostly in Aberdeen. This was completed on a unique welding machine. The company had run into financial difficulties and I acquired the venture at a good price with David Harrod, a businessman I knew from Aberdeen.

The company had its ups and downs with cashflow. We received a repossession order for our friction welder; it had been sold to another company because of a missed hire purchase payment. The following day I accompanied my lawyer to the High Court in Edinburgh and applied for an Administration Order to keep creditors at bay. The Administration Order was granted, giving us time to either sell the business, or trade out of the problem without creditor pressure – which we achieved.

We needed to buy new steel pipe for the business, and the preferred manufacturer was a company in Tokyo. En-route we stopped off in New York and San Francisco. We also visited Hawaii, where we stayed at the famous Pink Palace Hotel on Waikiki Beach. The tiny Hacienda-style hotel sits between skyscrapers on the shore.

From Hawaii we flew to Narita Airport, followed by a long and traffic-jammed bus ride into Tokyo. Once we arrived there, the hotel was a calm oasis amidst the city's hectic streets, with endless staff – including kimono-dressed women to bow us in and out of lifts – and clientele of every nationality.

On our first night in Tokyo, a representative of the Japanese company met us at the hotel for drinks and dinner. We went through to the elegant dining room, which had a rich red carpet and black-lacquered wood and more kimono-clad women bowing and serving the guests. It soon became clear that the man's business expenses allowed him to match us drink for drink – which he was very much encouraging us to do – and he had a taste for whisky! As the evening wore on – and his whisky tab mounted – we talked about almost everything other than steel pipes. That is the Japanese custom for conducting business.

Early the following morning, David and I were picked up on schedule after breakfast and taken to the factory where the pipe was manufactured. Our dining companion from the evening before introduced us to the company's executives, and then showed us around the factory.

We were taken to a room with elaborate decorations and given handle-less cups, full of steaming tea. Then the negotiations began – or rather our attempts at them, as their executives relentlessly kept to the quoted price.

As soon as we had come to an agreement, they insisted that we should all go to lunch at a special Tokyo restaurant. On arrival, we were shown to a private room with a single round table and the six of us were seated. The company president then told us there was only one dish on the menu that day, Kobe beef, which is a Japanese delicacy. It is considered the most exclusive beef in the world, renowned for its flavour, tenderness and fatty, well-marbled texture, achieved through constant massaging. It is certainly the most expensive, costing eye-watering amounts per pound. It tasted delicious and we felt honoured to have been served the delicacy and thanked our hosts graciously, as – negotiations aside – we had been treated so courteously.

We were taken back to our hotel, having made arrangements to meet up with our whisky-drinking friend later that evening at a restaurant in the downtown district. We made our way there by subway, slightly conscious of being taller than everyone else – albeit I am only 5'7". The streets were so clean and noticeably free from chewing gum. The pavement menace is sensibly banned from being consumed in public in Japan.

I was expecting a mass of frenetic people. Instead there were orderly lines of commuters following marked paths and none of the pushing and shoving that often happens elsewhere. We found the restaurant and our friend who was already enjoying a whisky. We were enthralled when he told us that Tokyo was home to thirty-five million people; commuters slept in tiny – air-conditioned spaces the size of cupboards; and there were too many rules and hilarious signs. He also told us all about the two hundred miles per hour bullet train.

The following afternoon we returned to the airport to catch our flight home. Although I was travelling in first class, I didn't want to sleep. Instead, I took in the view flying over the Arctic. I was not disappointed as snow and ice gradually replaced the green land beneath us; soon the mountains appeared to reach up to the plane. It was an amazing sight, and I felt privileged to have seen it. We landed back at Heathrow after travelling round the world in seven days, which was a first for me. We had achieved what we set out to do for the business and had an incredible adventure at the same time.

Back in Jersey, Sue had moved into my apartment. I had a houseful of ladies when the girls arrived for their holidays. My daughters adored Sue, as I did, because she was so genuine and thoughtful. For Sue's twenty-first birthday I wanted to arrange something special, so I secretly invited her twin Julie and her partner Phil down from Cumbria.

Sue was absolutely astonished when they turned up at the Grand Hotel. They were booked in as Mr and Mrs Smith as, of course, Sue was in charge of making reservations! We had a wonderful few days together, with a fair amount of champagne drunk and fantastic food eaten. And every time my daughters arrived from Aberdeen, the four of us would have fun together – on the beach, in the town, or simply watching TV at home.

One evening we had a brilliant time listening to Frank Sinatra's 'New York, New York', miming to the music, with me staggering around in Sue's shoes and laughing, just for the sake of it.

Then in 1986, I took Vicky to Monaco to celebrate her sixteenth birthday. On the flight out we travelled in Club Class. The cabin was empty except for the two of us and Benny Hill, who sat close by, looking petrified and avoiding eye contact. He seemed incredibly shy and so uncomfortable at having been recognised that I dared not approach him for an autograph; the contrast between his screen persona and what we saw could not have been greater. As we took off, Vicky passed me one of the headphones on her Sony Walkman, blasting out Dire Straits' 'Money for Nothing', her favourite album at that time.

We stayed in a sensational twin room at the Grand Hotel with views across the sea and relaxed at the rooftop pool. We also enjoyed walks around the port and shopping in Nice, visited the

Cafe de Paris, and had dinner while watching the Moulin Rouge-style show at The Grand Hotel. We received disapproving looks from people who clearly failed to see that my young companion was, in fact my daughter, and not an inappropriate youthful girlfriend. People would mutter comments that we could both hear, or point, or simply look at us, horrified. Vicky played up to this and learned to wait for a suitable moment to loudly call me 'Dad'. It was hard not to laugh at the look of relief on concerned faces, shortly followed by shame when people realised that they had assumed the worst.

In April 1987, Sue and I drove up to Cumbria to visit some of her family. We were out having a drink in her home town of Ulverston when my mobile phone rang.

'I have terrible news,' Dad told me when I answered the brick-sized, crackly Motorola device. 'Your mum has died.'

I couldn't speak. I was shocked. I cried. Her unhappy life flashed through my mind. What a waste. She was only fifty-five.

Mum had been ill – at times very seriously – for the past three years; in fact, she had not been well for decades, though we hadn't realised the extent of her problems for a long time. But, even at twelve, I knew that it wasn't right for mum to drink almost neat vodka as she prepared for a rare night out.

However, it was only much later, when I left home, that I realised how bad my mum's drinking had become. The root of it all was depression. Unfortunately her alcoholism escalated to such an extent that she was drinking two bottles of spirits and smoking sixty cigarettes a day.

Aged fifty-two, she'd had a heart attack and was unconscious for six months. Remarkably, Mum regained consciousness and never drank or smoked again. Clearly, though, substantial damage had already been inflicted. Three years later she had another, though less severe, heart attack. As she recovered from that setback in hospital, she suffered a further heart attack. Tragically, this time, she could not be resuscitated.

The funeral was a bleak affair. Few people other than family attended, and I felt an overwhelming sadness that, for most of my mum's life, happiness had been so elusive to her. For quite a few years prior to her death, I'd been sending her £150 each month, but much of it was found, unspent, in a bank account soon after her funeral. It seemed so sad that she had died so young and so unhappy.

Eventually, when I had worked through those feelings, I gained some acceptance in the realisation that opportunities – be they for fun, love, adventure or business – are to be seized as they come along in life. Yesterday has gone. All we have is today.

That year I travelled to Lafayette, Louisiana, where I'd invested in a tool company. The firm had invented a computerised lathe producing precision down-hole equipment for the oil industry. It was Jack Pillow's home town; however, I was there for another reason. The company was underperforming and my appearance, miraculously, prompted a turnaround.

I also started making regular trips to Houston with a fellow entrepreneur who was planning to open an office there for his drilling and pipe business. I was travelling with American Airlines first class so regularly that I became friends with some of the crew. Amy, a first class stewardess, lived in Pensacola, the most western town in the Florida Panhandle. Her father was the mayor and owned a unique bar, McGuire's Irish Pub. [6] The bar had a terrific ambience, with antiques and Tiffany lamps. Its ceiling was adorned with thousands of dollar bills, signed by Irishmen from all over the world.

Through McGuire, I learned of an apartment for sale for only $45,000 on Pensacola Beach, on the peninsula that stretches for miles into the Gulf of Mexico. It was a fabulous

6   The pub professes to now have over 750,000 dollar bills pinned to its ceiling and walls. It also has a large stuffed moose head mounted near the music stage and first-time visitors are encouraged to kiss it when they enter the pub!

location, and with the best beach of pure, fine white sand that I have ever seen. I had to buy it.

Unfortunately, I was so busy that I only managed to visit the property once. I decided to sell the place...I wonder who enjoys that gem of an apartment now?

CHAPTER SIX

Family Comes First

At my brother's home in Peckham Rye, preparing for bone marrow transplant.

At my brother's house in Peckham Rye, the alarm on my phone says 7 a.m. as I slowly stretch out of my pill-induced sleep. After my scheduled bone marrow transplant gave way to the removal of a kidney stone last month, the day has arrived for me to return to St George's for the procedure to finally begin. Chemotherapy is the first part of the process (this is called conditioning) to destroy the diseased cells in my bone marrow – and that begins tomorrow.

By 8 a.m. I'm showered and dressed and have worked my way through my morning doses from among the eight different medications – Ciprofloxacin, Fluconazole, Tamsulosin, G-CSF, Penicillin, Itraconazole, Desferal and Phenytoin. I have all of these to stop infections, reduce iron levels, and prevent fits. A taxi arrives promptly at 9 a.m. and, since the schools have all broken up for the summer, the traffic is light and I arrive in good time at the Ruth Myles Unit at St George's Hospital.

I know everyone at reception and they all greet me warmly and sense my delight when I'm told I have Room 3 again. The room was mine for the transplant ten years ago and also for my kidney stone removal. I take this as a good omen for the transplant.

There are thirteen rooms on the ward, five of which are isolation, with special one-way Hepa air filtration. Room 3 – with its window to the outside and another on to the main ward hospital corridor and central office station – seems to be the best of those. It's not yet ready, but I've arranged with Dara Qadir, the registrar/transplant fellow, to officially check in mid-afternoon as I'm meeting an old friend for lunch. My case is put into storage and I head off to the tube station.

It's a hot summer's day and I make my way across London's underground until I emerge in Knightsbridge besides Harrods. I've promised granddaughters Isla and Megan a small surprise for being good, and head to Beauchamp Place where there's an array of shops. I walk the entire street and near the end find a beautiful store selling bespoke cards and stationery. I choose two hand-printed cards that are suitable for six-year old girls. Once I'm back in hospital I'll write out the cards and put £10 in the ones for Isla and Megan as a holiday treat.

With time to spare I walk over to a nearby coffee shop and sit in the sun drinking a small latte, watching the world go by, and thinking of all the wonderful things in my life. Before long I see my friend David Rondel walking along the road. He has invited me to San Lorenzo, the iconic Italian restaurant. We spend a great couple of hours laughing and reminiscing about our decades-long friendship, and the trips we've made together for business and pleasure all across Europe and the States. Then it's time for me to retrace my steps and return to St George's Hospital for 4 p.m. as promised.

July 2rd 2014; day one at St George's Hospital, London.

Back in Room 3 I start to unpack. A nurse arrives to take my blood pressure and check my pulse and temperature. This routine will happen every four hours for the next five or so weeks.

Next come two nebulisers – both to prevent pneumonia – and the electrocardiogram (ECG) to check my heart activity, plus another round of pills: Ursodeoxycholic acid, Phenytoin, folic acid, Zorivax, Ondansetron and Domperidone.

The Hickman Line, which has remained in me since it was inserted prior to my kidney stone procedure, is flushed with a cleaning solution. I have a ham sandwich, a tomato and yoghurt for tea. Then, relaxed, I listen to music, call my brother David and chat to my daughters on Face Time.

In the early hours of the following morning I'm still awake, reliving what has been a very special day, and finally succumb to taking my sleeping pill.

July 24th 2014; day two at St George's Hospital, London.

The door to my room opens at 6 a.m., four hours since the last trio of blood pressure, temperature and pulse readings; it's the start of my first full day back in Room 3. I'm still feeling sleepy at 7.30 a.m. when I'm given a tiny paper cup with eight pills of assorted colours and sizes: Aciclovir, Folic Acid, Omeprazole, Caphasol, Ondansetron, Domperidone, Phenytoin and Ursodeoxycholic Acid.

By 8 a.m. I've showered and dressed when a breakfast of cornflakes, toast and tea arrives. Later in the morning Dr Mickey Koh, the consultant haematologist and the clinical lead for stem cell transplantation at St George's Hospital, comes in to talk about my case.

In the isolation room I feel like an island, set apart from all but my family, a few friends, and of course my donor, Axel, in Germany. I have plenty to keep me busy, including books and puzzles from my children. Technology has moved on so much since my last transplant and I now have an iPod, iPad and iPhone to pass the time.

To anchor myself through the transplant process I switch on my iPad and listen to two songs that connect me emotionally to my children. At the moment my life is metaphorically about getting from one side of a gorge to the other. These songs will inspire me when that journey gets tough and help me to the other side.

The one thing I have a choice about in this situation is my thought process. I will choose thoughts that are life affirming and not dwell on fear and create anxiety. Mind over matter.

The songs I have chosen to uplift me are Whitney Houston's 'One Moment In Time', and Martina McBride's 'In My Daughter's Eyes', which Louisa sent me and tells of a parent's love for a daughter. I immerse myself in both songs. I decide not to play the songs again, to keep emotions in check.

The nurses begin administering chemo at 4 p.m. The first dose is 204 mg of Busulphan, and three and a half hours later I receive 50 mg Fludarabine, with flushes in between. Both the Busulphan and Fludarabine are administered in saline solutions, and my daily fluid balance is measured in and out – and will continue to be – which is a chore, but essential. I've also had a line inserted that will slowly drip Heparin into my body for my entire stay. I am attached to a stand with a drip 24/7. However awkward this is, Heparin is an anticoagulant that prevents blood clots and is therefore vital during the procedure.

By then it's 8 p.m. and I'm told I'll receive a bag of platelets and a blood transfusion now, and another one in the morning. Between it all I manage to eat a cheese sandwich, some rice pudding and a banana. By 11.30 p.m. everything's completed and I take my sleeping pill for the night. I drift off, thinking about my childhood, so long ago, and yet so fresh in my mind.

★★★

I was almost born in a taxi on the way to hospital on 2 March 1951. The taxi just made it in time to Thorpe Hall, a beautiful Grade 1 listed mansion in Peterborough. The exquisite building, dating from the 17th Century, was used as a maternity hospital from 1947 until 1970. It has chocolate-box symmetry, pretty dormer windows, and elaborate architectural flourishes such as subtle frescos and a Tuscan pillared porch supporting a first-floor balcony. Even its gardens are sufficiently noteworthy to be listed, and it certainly provided an elegant setting for my entrance into this world.

My mother and I returned from Thorpe Hall to my paternal grandmother's house nearby in Peterborough, where my mother and father were living at the time with Gary, my elder brother. He had been born almost exactly a year before me on 11 March 1950. Grandmother Nan Evans had been a midwife. She was a warm and down-to-earth woman, yet also strong and single-minded.

My mother, Ruby, had been a rising ballet star, having been spotted aged eight for her potential, and sent to the Royal Ballet School in London to train. She landed the role as 'the legs' of Moira Lister when the actress played the Prima Ballerina in Michael Powell's classic film The Red Shoes, and later on she danced at the Windmill Theatre. She was certainly tipped for stardom until pregnancy and then a hasty marriage to my father; finally the birth of Gary compelled her into an early retirement.

Her father, Sidney Nicholls – who provided my middle name – worked as a cobbler out of his garden shed, having lost a leg while fighting in World War 1. He was certainly not well physically, because in addition to having lost his leg, which troubled him for the rest of his life, 'he'd had three heart attacks. Consequently, he was often depressed. He actually felt a lot of pain in the remains of the leg he had removed. Tragically, it seemed to those around him that he never escaped the horrors of World War 1. How could any soldier erase those memories, especially with a crippled body at a young age?

Sadly, Mum's personality also seemed to err towards

depression. This was perhaps a consequence of her disappointment of a lost career, or possibly as a result of the trauma of her dad committing suicide in the shed when she was fifteen. Perhaps it was a combination of the two.

My father, also Eric, was born at the very end of 1925 in Merthyr Tydfil, South Wales, giving me my 'taffy' roots. His own childhood had not been an easy one. He'd had a younger brother, Sonny, who'd died from diphtheria at the age of five. My dad's father had walked out on the family, leaving my grandmother to cope entirely on her own. From then on his childhood was quite lonely. I always wondered if that was the cause of his ambivalent feelings towards me.

Both of my parents were exceptionally good looking; my father, an architect, was classically handsome and my mother unquestionably beautiful. They made a picture-perfect couple. However, they were both reserved by nature and, although they both clearly loved and did their best for us, they weren't affectionate. Our household wasn't an especially happy one. My parents weren't sociable and we led a very isolated existence with virtually no visitors, and neighbours only spoken to over the garden fence. Only occasionally, other children came to play with us. There was zero chance of any sleepovers.

This may have been the result of our parents simply repeating their own emotionally stifled upbringing, or possibly a reflection of their marriage. Theirs was not a particularly happy union, it appeared to me, but then our mother was not a particularly happy woman. She had suffered continual loss over the years – her father by suicide, the end of her much loved ballet career, and then the tragedy of miscarrying twins late in pregnancy. That event shocked us all. I can still recall, in harrowing detail, the horror of her shocking blood-loss. I remember the look of despair on my father's face and the urgency of the ambulancemen. It is little wonder that my parents both struggled with life after that episode.

She must have also missed her sister, Pearl, who had moved to the States with her husband, Ray, an American Air Force Pilot from Canada. He'd been based at RAF Wittering near Peterborough and then returned home with his bride, but rarely came back to the UK for visits. Mum also had a brother, Reg, who served in the Tank Division during World War Two. His tank was the only one in his division to survive. Reg emerged from the hostilities with poor hearing after suffering the amplified noise of the bombs around him from the confines of his tank. He found work in a local hardwear store in Peterborough and married Cybil. I remember him as an easy-going man who loved reading comics, especially the Dandy and Beano.

Another of my earliest memories, and I must have been very young at the time, is showing a small girl how I was fixing my pride and joy – a red steel, single-seat pedal car with rubber wheels. On many levels, the mini motor was foreshadowing life ahead of me.

I was four years old when we moved from Nan Evans' house into our very own new home, designed by our dad in Francis Gardens, on the other side of Peterborough. It was open plan, single-story, L-shaped and modern for its time, and came with a garage and small garden. There were two bedrooms: one for my parents, and one for the boys.

On 9 May 1955, my younger brother David was born. He completed the trio of young Evans brothers in our bedroom.

Mum looked after us during the day until Dad returned from work at half-past five every evening, when they would head to the kitchen together. Dad tackled the cooking while mum chatted with him and had a drink of vodka. I'm not sure if this was because Dad really enjoyed cooking, or it wasn't mum's cup of tea.

After supper Dad would spend the evening watching TV – Coronation Street was one of many unmissable programmes – and that pattern rarely varied. Occasionally he played the saxophone and clarinet with a band he'd formed, and we had to keep out of the way. Unfortunately, I don't recall Mum having any interests of her own, but I imagine she was kept too busy looking after the house and all of us. She was a wonderful mother.

At home Dad took on the traditional role of being the family disciplinarian. I remember a vivid and painful event in my life. At the age of five or six I was punished for something I hadn't done. Whatever the supposed crime was, I don't remember; I only recall my mum trying to restrain my father. He dragged me into the garage and then bent me over a wooden trestle before hitting me six times on my backside with a paddle of wood. It was agony. I can still remember that. Despite this I never uttered a sound, not even when he asked me if I wanted more. He then hit me another three or so times for not answering.

I simply stood up and, with tears rolling down my face, walked away. I can still picture my mother sobbing when I returned to the kitchen after the beating. I also remember that, worse than the pain of the beating, was the feeling of indignation; my father had doubted my honesty. I lost a lot of respect for him that day, even if I did at least learn grit. I didn't speak to him for another week until he apologised after finding out that I had been telling the truth.

Dad, without knowing it, did me a huge favour. His appalling behaviour taught me to hide my feelings and take pain and pressure. I was learning how to cope with the incredible pressures that lay ahead in my life.

Sadly, the whole incident only served to widen the growing distance that was already emerging between the two of us. It was also, I now realise, a pivotal moment for defining how I would later deal with both physical and mental pain: by holding it in and not allowing my feelings to show. Perhaps this wasn't always the best approach.

Dad took Gary and me into Peterborough town centre on a Saturday morning while Mum stayed at home with David, until he was old enough to join us. We had a routine on those outings that seldom changed. There was the baker's shop, which I loved for its wonderful aroma of cakes and fresh bread. We bought a poppy-seed loaf or a French stick, custard slices and éclairs. At the model shop we'd browse, wide-eyed, at the kits or rows of model cars, trains and planes. The market offered fresh, local chickens, ready-plucked and waiting to provide a sumptuous Sunday lunch.

The market really fascinated me: the rabbits in cages waiting to be sold as pets or for food; likewise the baby chicks and full-grown chickens; the fruit, vegetable and flower stalls; and the stands selling tools or toys or clothing. In fact there were vendors selling just about anything. I could have walked around and watched the dealings all day; I became so mesmerised by it all that I'd end up getting lost in time. Certainly the process of buying and selling was evolving in my mind, even if I was not aware of it. In retrospect, these visits to the market confirmed my desire to be in business.

In 1956 I started at Fullbridge Road School, and used to walk there with Gary. On the way home, I played marbles with him in the gutter. I have few recollections from primary school, other than an incident when I was slightly older. Our form teacher, Mr C., was a sadist – and worse. He divided the class so that boys were on one side and girls on the other.

He'd pick on the boys and touch up the girls. It was hideous, and if he were a teacher today he would almost certainly be arrested. He had a two-foot long cane, and I was thrashed on several occasions for no reason at all. One boy was dragged by this maniac into a stockroom and caned until one of our classmates ran off to seek help.

We finally managed to put an end to his reign of terror when he left the cane behind on his desk. One of the boys (who could that be?) stole it – by slipping the despised piece of wood up his sleeve. The offending timber was duly cut into small pieces using a hacksaw, after which the segments were handed out like loot to those who had suffered at his hands. For a long time Mr C. did his best to intimidate us into revealing what had happened to his cane, but we never let slip the truth. Interestingly, he never replaced the missing cane.

From an early age I was fascinated by business and the whole process of buying, selling and negotiating. Perhaps in some way this stemmed from a desire to earn my parents' affections as I yearned to be hugged, cuddled or kissed by them. So it's possible that, in my longing for their love, I thought I could literally earn it; and if not their love, then at least my father's approval, which I craved equally. At any rate, finding ways to make money held magnetism for me and I believe I have a natural instinct for business.

At around five or six years old, no doubt also inspired by my weekly visits to Peterborough market, I opened a 'shop' in my bedroom.

My mother would lend me money to buy variety packs of cereal and tea, along with coffee and multi-coloured snowdrop sweets. I would then sell to my mother or my brothers. I would repay my mother's loan out of the profit. Sometimes she would buy a packet of Frosties for my breakfast, which I would leave uneaten in order to sell them back to her the next day. At the time I thought it was a great idea, but looking back I realise I was hardly being fair to my mum. It was good of her to indulge me in this way and I absolutely loved the process, which was far more than a mere game to me, but the beginning of a passion. I have my mother to thank for my induction into business at five years old.

My future self as a tough negotiator also came to the fore in the unlikely sphere of the Cub Scouts. I joined the Cubs when I was eight, mainly because I knew I could get chips and scraps on the way home after the meeting with the weekly thrupenny bit pocket money from my dad.

Having joined, it was the Bob-a-Job week that brought out my inner Gordon Gekko. It transpired like this: I knocked on a door and the owner said he would pay me to collect clay pots for his greenhouse; I asked him how many and he replied, 'As many as you can get'. I spent four hours calling at every house in the neighbourhood, after which I had collected around thirty pots of all shapes and sizes.

I was excited at the prospect of showing the man what I'd achieved, and he was certainly surprised when he saw how many I'd brought round. He then put his hand in his pocket and produced a shilling. He asked for the green and yellow sticker to put in his window to show he'd taken part in Bob-a-Job week. I was furious. I told him that I thought my efforts were worth at least 12/6 (twelve shillings and six pennies) and had planned on keeping the difference! We couldn't agree a figure and he threatened to report me, while I accused him of abusing the Cubs.

It was not a dignified exchange or a happy outcome for either of us: the man didn't get his pots, I didn't get the money I'd hoped for and he did indeed report me to the Cubs. I ended up with a severe telling off from Akela.

However, it taught me some valuable lessons – not to be greedy or to push the limits in situations. But, looking back, it also shows that I would go – both literally and figuratively – the extra mile to be successful.

Even before the age of ten, I was highly ambitious and always on the lookout for an opportunity to expand my money-making schemes beyond the confines of the bedroom shop.

One day, when I was about seven, my father asked me what I wanted to be when I grew up. In all seriousness I answered that I wanted to be a millionaire and drive a gold Rolls Royce with my personal number plate. My dad laughed, but patronisingly, which upset me deeply.

In that moment he cemented the goal so strongly into my spirit that it was as if the deed was already done – I just didn't have the date or exact method.

I began doing a paper round each morning before school and again on a Sunday. The Sabbath editions were so heavy that I couldn't ride my bike until the half-way stage. After that I would visit all the houses to collect the week's paper money. Some mean residents tried to fob me off, but I persevered as a mini debt collector and always secured the proceeds of my daily endeavours.

By age nine I was also working on the fruit and veg stall at the town market in Peterborough, earning 17/6 for the day.

I'd arrive at 6.30 a.m. to unload the lorry, set up the stall and then work happily for twelve hours. I'd have one break in the day when I would buy a Wimpy hamburger or fish and chips, which I ate under the stall. On those Saturdays I was probably the happiest boy in town.

Later on, when the market moved to new premises, I worked on a stall selling tools. After that I moved to another fruit and vegetable stall, where my earnings rose to eighteen shillings for the day. Unfortunately, my father, who was a bit of a snob, was always appalled by the idea of his son working at the market. In addition I washed four cars for £1 on Sundays – good money in those days. I was always more of a saver than a spender, but I did treat myself to a record player as well as The Beatles' Hard Day's Night and an album by Neil Sedaka.

By that age we were taking annual holidays, venturing in our maroon and silver Triumph Mayflower to nearby popular resorts. We visited Clacton-on-Sea in Essex, or Mundesley, a pretty village on the Norfolk coast, plus Skegness, the famous seaside town in Lincolnshire. We also travelled to Gorleston, a traditional holiday resort on the mouth of the River Yare in south Norfolk. I have happy memories of those holidays, apart from the tortuous journeys there and back with my father stressing out behind the wheel of our car.

Gary, David and I were always excited at the prospect of our holidays away. The night before, when the suitcases came out, we'd stay up late talking through our plans for the beach. We'd always be up early, dressed and ready to go while our parents whiled away the morning with last-minute packing and endless debates about what – and what not – to take. Eventually the boot would be loaded and then Gary, David and I would pile inside the old Triumph. Dad wedged in extra bags and cases and a light blue potty with a handle, to relieve us of the necessity for loo breaks! By the time everything was crammed in – including buckets, spades, fishing rods, and deck chairs, as well as a full picnic for the journey – we looked like we were going on safari.

No doubt some of these stories will resonate with older readers and remind you of holiday memories with your parents. We all carry the child that grew up to an adult inside us...

We all cheered when we finally left our road and pulled

onto the main street. As we left Peterborough and the 30mph speed limit, Dad accelerated up to a breathtaking 35mph. He maintained this breakneck speed for the entire journey while, for some unknown reason, driving on the cat's eyes in the centre of the road. The noise and shuddering was awful – as was the reaction from other drivers.

Oncoming vehicles blasted their horns at us, as did overtaking trucks and cars. But Dad appeared oblivious to the inconvenience he was causing. Before long he would be demanding a sandwich or a sweet and soon a neck massage from Mum.

I remember when Gary needed to pee and asked if we could stop the car for his call of nature.

'Tell him to use the potty!' he instructed Mum; Dad had a rule that we were not allowed to talk directly to him while he was driving.

'The car's moving around too much and I can't keep the potty still!' wailed Gary.

'We can't stop!' Dad insisted.

Gary was squealing with frustration but forced to use the potty, leaving David and me in hysterics at the unfolding pantomime. Necessities done, Gary handed the potty to mum who opened the car window and gingerly emptied it when no other vehicle was nearby.

Shortly afterwards we stopped as Dad needed a break, and our parents shared a flask of tea while the three of us let off some steam. Rest over, we all piled back in the car and our epic journey continued at its previous snail's pace. Boredom was getting the better of us, and we could only pass the time by being silly, mimicking being sick in the potty, or pretending to need to pee.

Then Gary did actually need to pee again and, after another round of backseat acrobatics, he carefully handed the potty with its unstable cargo to my mother. She made a vain attempt to throw the contents out of the moving car. For whatever reason, Mum had forgotten to open the window and the pee exploded through the car like a champagne bottle opening. Everyone, including Dad, received a good soaking. Neither Gary, David nor I could contain ourselves; we thought it was hilarious. Our irritable driver continued on the painful journey in a complete rage.

Finally, after taking around seven hours to cover about a hundred miles, which the rest of us knew was ridiculously long, we'd reach our destination. Once at the resort, we'd stay in either a bed and breakfast guest house, or rent a caravan, and my brothers and I would finally have some fun together. We enjoyed all the traditional activities of a British seaside holiday – playing on the beach, taking donkey rides while enjoying doughnuts, popcorn and ice-cream. These are some of my happiest memories of us all being together as a family. The only dread that we had was the return journey – along the same route and lasting just as long.

Christmas, and the build-up to the big day, was another exciting time. Each year the Christmas decorations would come down from the attic in their various boxes. Dad took charge while the whole family decorated the Christmas tree – usually at the last minute – with tinsel and plastic ice sticks and small animals in snow. Best of all were the rainbow-coloured paper chains, looped together and then laced across the house. December always seemed to go so slowly, but as the days went by our excitement grew.

Come Christmas Eve, Mum and Dad would be in a panic over all the last minute preparations, with Dad doing most of the cooking. Gary, David and I would go to bed and, on Christmas morning wait patiently at the top of the stairs with the smell of the pine tree and special food whetting our excitement. Only when our parents were ready – never early on the big day – were we allowed downstairs to open our presents. Soon after that both Nan Evans and Nan Nichols would arrive to have lunch with us all – this was the only day Nan Evans ever came to visit – and afterwards we would all gather around the tiny black and white TV. We watched the usual Christmas fare, and for New Year I remember Andy Stewart and his kilted guests dancing around in the White Heather Club.

My most memorable recollection of Christmas is from when I was around ten or eleven. I'd decided to buy Mum and Dad a set of crockery. I looked around the market and found an attractive willow pattern. I bought it piece by piece with my earnings each week. I began in September and by Christmas I'd bought six each of dinner plates, side plates, cereal bowls, cups and saucers, two large serving plates and a milk jug and tea pot.

They had no idea what I was up to. I was so proud of my efforts and carefully wrapped each piece before packing them in a sturdy box, covered in silver paper and a ribbon from Woolworths.

That Christmas morning I struggled downstairs carrying two boxes, full of excitement and looking forward to handing over festive treats to Mum and Dad. Unfortunately their response was muted, at best. They seemed overwhelmed at how much there was to open and patiently unwrapped every item – but their apparent lack of enthusiasm felt devastating. However, my disappointment on that day was eventually replaced by the realisation that the crockery was, in fact, used at every meal for years afterwards. To this day I prefer to give rather than to receive.

When I was eleven we moved to a larger, newy-built house in Audley Gate, not far from Thorpe Hall where I was born. Unknown to my parents I went into a newsagent in the new shopping precinct nearby and asked if I could have a job, initially stocking the shelves and then serving at the counter. The idea of helping this new enterprise as it opened for business excited me greatly. I loved the whole process of filling the shelves and taking the money.

Opposite the newsagent's was a small supermarket whose owners' son was a friend of mine. One day he told me that he could get the key to the stockroom, which he boasted was always full, and we could take what we wanted without ever being found out. Of course this sounded something of a paradise to my young ears. When my friend did in fact get the key we gleefully took a carton of Benson and Hedges, a box of Swan Vestas matches, and a large box containing several packets of Maltesers. We stuffed our haul into a suitable bag and sneaked out of the newsagents, along a railway line behind the store, over a stile and into a wheat field that led to a small clearing of trees and a high-banked stream.

It was a glorious summer's day with the wheat, almost ready to be harvested, swaying in the wind. We sat down under a small tree on the edge of the wheat field, opened the first box of chocolates and just helped ourselves, laughing without any thought of our actions. Then we did the same with the cigarettes and matches. I'd never smoked before and puffed my way unenthusiastically through two, but couldn't face any more after that. We then wondered how we'd get rid of the evidence and decided that the best solution would be to burn everything. The fire started easily, and we soon added all the cartons, unsmoked cigarettes, and boxes of matches.

We were thrilled with our ingenuity; the fire reminded us of Bonfire Night as the matches produced a shower of sparks. But then suddenly the tree above us was on fire too and, before we could react, the wheat field was alight. My friend and I could only watch in horror as the wind quickly swept the fire across the wheat. We decided to run to the very bottom of the field, several hundred yards away, where the stream's high bank hid us from view and the fire couldn't spread any further.

A train passed by and we just bobbed under the bank so we couldn't be seen, and then our horror grew as we heard sirens approaching.

First came the fire engines, six in total, and then the police shortly afterwards. As the wind whipped the flames in all directions the fire engines spread around the field in a desperate attempt to grasp control of the growing nightmare. The smell of the burning wheat was awful, but we stayed rooted to our spot, terrified at the thought of the consequences.

By and by, as the fire came under control, we looked at the devastation we'd caused. The field of wheat was gone and in its place was black smoking earth with a clear view to the road to our front, the railway track to our left, and the line of trees to our right. Frightened and anxious to escape, as well as put the shameful episode behind us, we eventually stood up and walked along the bank close to the stream. We were less likely to be seen on the way back to our separate homes. Our guilty secret was never discovered, even though the story was splashed across the local newspapers.

However, we didn't get away from the day's events entirely scot free as my friend's parents discovered that their stock had gone missing. They confronted their son, who confessed to that part of our misdemeanour. I was called in to face a severe telling off and to receive my punishment: working in their small supermarket, filling shelves and serving customers. Little did they realise that, to me, this was something of a treat. Furthermore, they didn't even tell my parents.

Another fond memory from my childhood is our annual

family visit to the fair in the centre of Peterborough. I recall our growing excitement as we crested the bridge over the River Nene and the distant coloured lights of the rides came into view against the darkening evening sky. After we parked our car and walked closer, our ebullience added to the crescendo of sound from excited people and heavy duty fairground engines.

The wafts of trampled summer grass, and diesel mixed with the sweet treats of candyfloss, toffee apples and doughnuts as well as the savoury smells of fried onions and hot dogs, all made for an irresistible mix. My everlasting memory is the scent filling the balmy air, the simple pleasure of eating a toffee apple, and a wistful backward glance as we drove home over the bridge. Older readers may well share those vivid fairground memories.

The lights and sounds faded into the distance, and we knew that we'd have to wait another year to return to the fair.

Soon after I entered my teens, my father decided that I should be sent off to boarding school. I was struggling academically at the local school in Peterborough and, despite my best efforts to learn, my reports were full of comments such as 'he tries but hasn't quite got a grip of this subject' and 'a keen and conscientious pupil'. My attempts to pass exams always appeared to be in vain, and before too long the reality of a succession of failed exams meant that I hated school.

My father thought that sending me away to the Royal Wolverhampton School would teach me discipline and provide much desired 'O' levels. He sent me away with the best of intentions. I wasn't so sure.

I can still remember the feeling of desolation after being left on the steps at my new school, waving goodbye to Mum and Dad for the first time at the age of fourteen. We'd gone to the cinema the evening before and watched the Sound of Music – my first ever visit to see a film. Somehow the closeness of the von Trapp family only highlighted the feeling of separation from my own parents.

The trunk was about my size and weight, and I knew none of the three hundred boys aged from six to eighteen. My sheltered existence was lost overnight in my brutal introduction to 'the real world'. I felt profoundly alone being so far from home, and I certainly felt unloved. My feelings about boarding school never improved and, without exception at the end of every holiday, I dreaded going back. It was really hard meeting new people at the age of fourteen and trying to make new friends in an unfamiliar place.

The Royal Wolverhampton School originally cared for orphans in 1850, following the cholera epidemic that had swept through England the year before. By the 1940s it had evolved into a government funded private school for boys whose fathers had been killed in the war. During the year I joined, fee-paying boys were admitted for the first time at a cost of £365 annually. The change had been a controversial one within the school, and there was a distinct division between the two groups of boys – the fee-paying and non-fee-paying. The atmosphere could become hostile.

I hated just about everything at boarding school. I detested the cold winters in unheated buildings and the stench of urine and vomit that could never be washed out of the wooden floors in my dorm. The food was horrible. Scanty trays of buns and chips were handed out, with never enough to go round. Powdered milk on our cornflakes was never properly mixed, so that the powder exploded while you ate the cereal.

I hated the narrow steel beds, curtains hung in windows at the front of the building but not at the back; the uniform which, barring the long black, yellow and red scarf was awful; the service every morning at the church within the school grounds and then a longer two-and-a-half hour endurance test on hard wooden benches every Sunday. I was bullied, trapped and desperately lonely.

The bullying – verbal, emotional and physical – was beyond belief, particularly towards the small boys, of which I was one. I witnessed and experienced all the tribulations that one associates with a boys' boarding school: fagging; sexual advances between pupils; and inappropriate behaviour by teachers towards pupils. One boy became so desperate to get away from the teacher in question that he set fire to the library in order to get expelled – a ploy that worked.

I was also desperately homesick for my brothers, who attended day schools back in Peterborough, and I missed the comforts and freedom of home life. I said nothing to my father as I knew, instinctively, that my complaints would fall on deaf ears. I felt locked in and trapped, as if I had been sent to prison.

Everything at school was regulated including getting up, washing, eating, doing prep, playing sport and writing letters

On Sunday afternoons, we went for a walk in our school uniforms. Another older boy and I would take eight smaller pupils out for two to three hours.

We went to bed at 8.30 p.m. The only unregulated events were short breaks in the morning, afternoon and before evening prep. There was also an hour a week when we could watch TV before bed.

For much of the time I lived for the refuge and comparative tranquillity of my bed, where I could hide under the sheets and blanket and to an extent switch off; with so many boys in the dorm that was hard to do. Some boys found solace through cricket and football on Saturday afternoons. For me, it contained the prospect of even more bullying and failure.

Aside from half-term, there were only two Exeats – for three hours on a Saturday afternoon. Dressed in school uniform, I'd walk into Wolverhampton on my own, past the Molineux football ground to look at the shops and perhaps even visit Beaties, the local department store. We had no freedom and were not allowed out unless under strict instruction and, or, control: the only time I felt free was when I was heading away from the school for an Exeat outing, half-term, or at the end of term for the school holiday. It's a shame that I was too young to comprehend that freedom is, more than anything, a state of mind.

Dad had to borrow money to send me to boarding school, which I didn't know at the time. I now really appreciate the sacrifice he made for me. I longed for letters, but only my mum made contact, while I wrote home with whatever news I had during the compulsory letter writing time each week; phone calls either to or from home were forbidden.

For two years I lived for the school holidays, Christmas in particular, and the day when I would leave at sixteen. The anticipation increased as it became ever more apparent I would never get the 'O' levels that were so important to Dad. This was in spite of my best efforts; from the very first day at the school I had promised myself that I would concentrate and work hard at all times. My mission was to achieve as many 'O' levels as possible.

The lack of academic improvement was clearly not for my lack of trying, as even more reports stated: 'Eric tries but he has not quite got a grip on this subject', 'Eric works as hard as ever', 'Aims very high', or 'Keen' – however, my grades showed irrevocably that I was not, and would never be, an academic achiever.

Much to my disappointment and embarrassment I didn't pass my mock 'O' levels and was told that I wouldn't be allowed to take the actual exams. The school didn't want my anticipated poor results showing in their records. I was so distraught with the news that one night I broke out of school and phoned home in tears, begging my father to collect me. Of course he adamantly refused to do that, which I should have expected,

'I paid for you to be there,' he muttered. 'You'll stay there. I'll collect you when all the other boys leave.'

And that was that.

I never received any accolade from my father. The agony of being treated like that had a profound effect on me; it drove me to the point of perfection with effort and time in any business. Having never achieved qualifications or enjoyed school. I was desperate to do something I wanted and liked – and I knew the rewards would come my way.

Listening to music on one of the prefect's record players became my escape, in particular the Mamas and Papas song 'Monday Monday', which became my anthem for freedom. I loved The Beatles' LP 'Sgt. Pepper's Lonely Hearts Club Band' and played the record endlessly. My mood was also lifted by some high-spirited antics shortly before the Christmas term ended during my final year. Four of us stole matron's knickers, took down the school flag at the front of the building, and hoisted up the purloined garments. We also lifted the maths teacher's new red Mini through the archway between the quadrangle and lawn, and squeezed it into the space between two flights of steps. The furious teacher had to recruit strong-armed colleagues to perform the same routine in reverse.

We weren't caught, although they were both close calls. Perhaps my most pleasant memory is the occasion when I accidentally grabbed matron's ample breast while running around the corner of a corridor. We both blushed. I fully expected to be either thrashed or expelled. However, nothing happened – although the matron smiled at me every time she saw me after this bizarre event.

Educationally, the only event of interest that I can recall was our local MP Enoch Powell giving a talk at our school. At the time his tirade about immigration seemed rather strange to us all. What would Mr Powell have said about modern Britain?

On the last day of term I packed my trunk for the final time, dragged it to the main hall and waited for my parents amidst the chaos. Three hundred other boys were equally excited at the prospect of going home at the end of another school year. After two years, enduring all that boarding school life had thrown at me, I was emerging with neither qualifications nor friendships: to all intents this sad episode in my life had been an expensive failure.

Now that I was finally leaving, I was so excited and hoping my dad would arrive early. The first car arrived at 9.30 a.m. and I watched the parents hug and kiss their son before heading off with him. Then 10.30 came and went, and then 11.30. Soon it was lunchtime and there were only two of us left at the school.

By 12.45 I was left completely on my own and the caretaker came to lock up the school. For four hours I had stared down the drive, yearning for my parents to arrive, with a growing sadness as every other boy left. For the next three-and-a-quarter hours I sat with the caretaker, feeling hurt and confused,

Finally, at 4 p.m., my parents eventually drew up. By then, I was no longer excited, just terribly disappointed. They hadn't even left the house in Peterborough at 9.30 a.m., when the first boy had already been collected.

I spent the next year at home in Peterborough, trying to scrape together those elusive five 'O' levels at the local Technical College. I just couldn't grasp Maths, English,

History Geography and Religious Instruction. Had they taught me business studies, I would have ended up running the school.

However, despite my best intentions and efforts – and I really was trying hard – after another year of endeavour, my only achievement was a cycling proficiency badge. I had failed school completely, and there was no point in continuing along the educational path.

Why did I fail so miserably at school? I believe I have slight dyslexia, although in those days there were no tests for that – or even any real interest in anyone other than the brightest and the best in each class.

I remember one incident in particular, standing in front of my class of thirty pupils, when I was eight years old. I had been instructed to read a passage of Kipling aloud to everyone. But the words came spluttering out, muddled and nonsensical, immediately followed by an eruption of cruel laughter from my classmates. I was mortified. Leaving school all those years later came as something of a relief, even if I had no qualifications and the employment exchange was my only next option.

But out of it all I did learn some valuable lessons, even if they were not the ones on the curriculum. Now, looking back, I do not think that I would have achieved all I did without those underlying lessons from boarding school.

From out of the sadness, the loneliness, the lack of support and any sense of direction, I gained the ability to be strong and never give up. I learned the value of having the freedom to make one's own choices in life, and that enabled me to work for myself rather than someone else.

I learned that, even though the terms passed so slowly, I could relive the excitement of going home over and over in my head. It made life at the school more tolerable.

Repeating these experiences over and over in my head has

trained my brain to vividly recall any memory – almost as if I was living it for the first time again.

I also learned that even the most painful situations can – with enough patience and a strong enough belief in the future – eventually be left behind.

CHAPTER SEVEN

Into Africa

Back at St George's Hospital, preparing for my bone marrow transplant.

My family is the most important part of my life. My hospital tests were punctuated by a wonderful few days in Norfolk with my daughter Vicky; my brothers Gary and David; David's partner Jeanette; and their daughter Sydney. Their love and support have reminded me how fortunate I am and what matters most in life. It was a very special long weekend, and I immersed myself in the emotional warmth that my family wrapped around me. Yet not far from my thoughts was the reality that this might be our last ever time together. Saying my goodbyes, especially to my daughter Vicky at Norwich Airport, was the hardest part; but that only emphasised all the reasons why I want to live and all that I have to look forward to on the other side of the transplant. Gary and I drove back down to London and a few days later David joined us, and my daughter Louisa flew in from France. I spent another superb few days with my two brothers and Louisa. Time zoomed past. Before I knew it, I was standing on the platform at London Bridge, blinking back tears while I watched Louisa's train become a distant dot as she left to return to Gatwick Airport. No matter their age, it seems that parting from one's children never gets easier.

July 25th 2014. Day three at St George's Hospital, London.

It's Friday, which at St George's is the day the entire team of specialist doctors and nurses make the rounds of patients. I've developed a rash over most of my body and am given a steroid cream to clear that up. Water retention has caused my feet and legs to swell up, for which I'm given medication that takes me from 71 to 68 kilos in two hours. Other than that, the medical team who visit me seem pleased with my progress.

I'm reminded from my last long stay in hospital that, the longer you're there, the less important time seems. Having said that, I am desperate to get better as quickly as possible. However, I cannot rush or speed up the process and instead I must simply let it be.

The key is to live fully in the atmosphere and routine of the isolation room. To help I have four photos of my family on the board beside my bed, everything that I brought in to keep me entertained, the hospital TV and of course my imagination. I use my mind to visualise myself wherever I choose. I just need to make certain that it's somewhere positive.

My chemo begins at 2 p.m. and is finished four hours later. Again I'm administered 204 mg of Busulphan and 50 mg Fludarabine, while the Hickman Line is flushed before, between and after use. I watch all the drips empty from the bag, grateful in the knowledge that these medicines are going to kill my remaining damaged bone marrow. When this is completed, I'm given a further bag of platelets. By mid-evening I'm feeling a little sick but am given another anti sickness pill, which helps, and I make myself eat a few crisps and a banana.

I had a visit from Suzanne Ruggles today. She is an amazing woman. I met her during my first transplant and subsequent check-ups back at the hospital in the months following the procedure; by the time I'd finished my post-transplant care, we'd become good friends.

Suzanne introduced supportive therapies to St George's Hospital *after being critically ill herself with a case of meningitis that took her to the brink of death. She even had the last rites administered.*

Following her recovery she sold her business and studied reflexology, health psychology and went to Harvard to study the science of relaxation techniques. She then managed, after much lobbying and her appointment in an administrative role at the hospital, to improve the lives of so many patients.

Inspired by her own journey and keen to help others, she founded the Full Circle Fund as a charity in 2006. I was happy to assist her with that, and also to donate £5,000 to the cause. The story of my first transplant case in 2004, which she found inspiring for my positive attitude and brevity of hospital stay, was written as a case study on the Full Circle website. I was named as a founding member.

Suzanne thought that if other patients could be supported to approach their illness in the way that I, and another similarly minded patient had done, it would be good for all concerned. In short, she felt there was so much that could be done from the core of the NHS to support a person facing the huge challenges of a life-threatening illness.

Her motto is: the person, first and always. The Full Circle Fund's mission statement is "to work hand-in-hand with conventional medicine to help support patients' physical recovery during and after treatment". The charity is self-financing in order that it remains beyond the vagaries of the NHS budget.

Today the Full Circle Fund Therapy Team is based in the haematology, paediatric and oncology wards of St George's. As I write, Full Circle is expanding into new spheres within the NHS, having been asked to provide their expertise for neuro-intensive care patients and for those undergoing neuro-rehabilitation. Their team of skilled therapists provide over 1,500 treatments a year to very sick babies, children and adults. Indeed, all through my visits for blood transfusions during these past months I've been fortunate enough to benefit from the charity's work. I've had reflexology while receiving blood each Monday, and I am now having regular treatments during this stay. As a result, when Suzanne came to see me today, we had a lot to talk about.

Later on in the evening I make Face Time calls to my family and catch up on emails from friends wishing me well. Speaking on Skype or Face Time is like having visitors, but without the strain of having to 'entertain' them when you feel awful, or the restrictions of visiting hours. By 11 p.m. I am in bed and drifting into another pill-induced sleep. My thoughts drift off to an African adventure.

★★★

On a cold and damp February afternoon in Edinburgh, a business contact offered me the opportunity of investing in Cape Palmas Logging – an old, well-established company in Liberia, West Africa. The company exported logs and sawn timber all over the world; however, for the past two years it had been poorly managed, and operations in both the bush and at its sawmill had ceased. As a result it had reached a financial crisis, with a huge debt owed to Liberia's Forestry Development Authority.

That said, it still retained its logging permit for 374,000 acres from the Liberian government, which had a further sixteen years to run, and its owner was part of the country's ruling elite.

Straight away, I was interested in the project. I had always been keen on a fresh business challenge as well as the chance to travel somewhere new, and this venture certainly ticked both of those boxes. Within weeks I had boarded a flight to spend five days in Liberia, checking out the company.

I'd been to Africa before – to Gabon a couple of times, and also to Cameroon – but even at the check-in at Heathrow there were signs of confusion and disorder. Liberia promised a new level in disorganisation. The plane stopped at Freetown in Sierra Leone and all but five people disembarked before we took off again for the short flight down to Monrovia, the capital of Liberia.

It was a daytime flight, with the blue-grey of the Atlantic Ocean clearly visible on one side of the plane and vast swathes of forests and mist-shrouded mountains on the other. As we came into land at Roberts International Airport, clusters of villages and smoke plumes from bonfires came into view.

The humidity hit me straight off the plane, but I'd coped with that before, so I wasn't too fazed. A small white building made do as the arrivals hall. Other planes had just landed and passengers began milling around.

Inside the building, people jostled and hauled bulging plastic bags and crammed cardboard boxes, or overflowing bags with broken zips. Many of these arrivals were, not too subtly, bribing the customs officers to jump the queues. The air was heavy with the fetid smell of perspiration. With all the pushing and shoving it took me an hour to exit the customs hall where, among the chaotic throng, I caught sight of a tall, distinguished figure. It could only be Lavoisier Tubman, the president of Cape Palmas Logging.

The airport was like nothing I'd seen or dealt with before – complete pandemonium. Hundreds of people formed a tangled swarm, and I was almost mobbed by the crowd, which felt quite intimidating. By this time I was the only white man left at the airport, and people were running and shoving around me trying to sell me whatever they could. I was offered a partly-used Bic pen and a tatty box of Swan Vestas matches. These were desperate people.

We pushed our way through the grasping crowd, keeping a tight hold of all possessions. Lavoisier was tall with a broad, kind smile and I immediately liked him.

He slapped me on the back with a grin and said: 'Welcome Eric, pleased to meet you. Let's get out of here.'

One detail I knew: Lavoisier's father, William Tubman, had been the President of Liberia from 1944 until his death, in a London clinic, in 1971.

As we climbed aboard Lavoisier's much-loved Mitsubishi Shogun, I told him that I was eager to know more about the country's history. His driver quickly slung my suitcase in the back, and then we set off through the horde towards Monrovia.

'I've never seen anything like this. Please tell me about Liberia,' I urged.

As Lavoisier's driver lurched the large 4x4 into gear, my companion smiled and began to chat in his American-educated accent.

'Liberia is Africa's oldest republic', he told me. 'The country was founded by freed American and Caribbean slaves. Many of our people are descended from the slaves.'

'How long ago did all this happen?' I asked, genuinely interested.

Lavoisier was in full flow: 'Yes, a colony was set up in Africa in the early 1800s. The first ship, Mayflower of Liberia, left New York on 6 February 1820. The American Colonization Society set up the first settlement, and it was known as Liberia. Independence was declared on 26 July 1847.'

He explained that his grandfather was one of around seventy slaves freed in America and sent to the Commonwealth of Liberia in 1844.

'And that is why I am here today,' he beamed. 'My father William was regarded as the father of modern Liberia. There was a military coup a few years ago, led by Samuel Doe. You could say that things have become fairly unstable since then.'

Lavoisier continued to give me a potted history with fact after fact, including Firestone's involvement with a million acres of rubber trees for tyre production.

'This country is so rich in natural resources. We have gold, silver, diamonds, iron ore and an infinite supply of timber. You will be impressed with this country's potential.'

It became immediately apparent that the country was badly run. On my visit to Gabon the country was clean and orderly with modern well-kept buildings, infrastructure and cars, and I had expected Liberia to be same; however, the contrast could not have been greater. Roads, buildings, vehicles and everything else seemed to be in a poor state of repair. There had been a total lack of investment in the country – and the place seemed to be completely out of control.

Roberts International Airport was around a forty-minute drive from Monrovia. It wasn't long before I caught my first glimpse of the forests from the ground. I could detect the unique, earthy smell of baking red soil and the drenched tropical vegetation.

Soon enough we entered the capital, with its narrow alleys snaking a path through the shanty towns and children playing on rubbish heaps. Finally the roads widened and we arrived in Sinkor, a more prosperous part of the city where Lavoisier lived with his wife Esther. The drive had been terrifying, with some of the most dangerous overtaking I had ever seen, and I was thankful to arrive at the house.

Lavoisier invited me into his study and spread out a sheaf of documents across a vast board table that dominated the room. One of his staff brought me black, sweet tea and I sat down to study the papers.

'These documents confirm the authenticity and assets of Cape Palmas Logging as a company,' he said, going through a number of records and reports while I read each one in turn.

We were interrupted by the door opening. A short, sharply-dressed woman walked in and strode towards us.

'My wife, Esther,' Lavoisier said, introducing us.

Lavoisier proved to be friendly, warm and welcoming. Esther was the complete opposite. She was plainly forceful – aggressive even – and I disliked her on sight. Her eyes were hard and she stared at me with open hostility. She stayed for the remainder of the proceedings, and contributed nothing other than animosity. But at least I learned where the power lay between them.

'Ok,' he said, when I'd finished looking through the paperwork, 'shall we take a plane out to the sawmill tomorrow?'

'I'm looking forward to it,' I replied eagerly.

We both stepped outside and clambered on board his Shogun once more. The driver set off through the chaotic streets for Le Meridien hotel, where I had booked a five-day stay.

I watched the crowds surging through the streets and around the car, with the women carrying all manner of goods on their heads. Children in ragged clothes kicked tin cans or ran alongside cars. The men, I noticed, just stood around chatting in clusters and smoking.

The hotel had a cordon of khaki-uniformed security guards, but once inside it seemed an oasis of calm after the mayhem of the city streets. As we approached the bar Lavoisier pointed out various businessmen, politicians and journalists along the way, as well as a couple of crooks. Liberia was certainly turning out to be a colourful country.

Our arrival at the bar caused quite a stir. Lavoisier was obviously well known. Soon, men began to approach us, one by one, each giving Lavoisier an eager handshake, and I could tell that he was well liked. And I could see why, as there was an air of undoubted grace and calm about the man.

When I finally reached my room I opened the window and heard, for the first time, the high pitched trill of the yellow-beaked and red-bellied mynah birds. I was exhausted and collapsed into bed, but could barely sleep for excitement. Despite the chaos of the place, my intuition told me that I could bring Cape Palmas Logging back into profit.

The next morning Lavoisier's lumbering vehicle came to collect me at half past six. At that hour the city was still cool and relatively quiet. It was an easy drive out of central

Monrovia to Spriggs Payne Airport, which serviced Liberia's domestic flights.

There, we met Quinca, a slim and elegant Spaniard who ran a tiny airline consisting of about five small planes, mainly on hire to the logging industry. Quinca pointed us towards a Cessna 172.

Within minutes the runway had been cleared of children playing football, and we headed south over a series of sandbars. Vast, dark waves from the Atlantic bore down on the shore. I could see the occasional boat and tiny figures of fishermen inside; the broad river coiled between trees to the ocean; and the mangrove swamps crouched menacingly between the land and the sea, sheltering perfect breeding grounds for mosquitoes.

As we followed the strip of palms down the coast for a couple of hours before turning inland towards the bush, Quinca listed some of the worst local health hazards: malaria, blackwater fever, yellow fever, leeches, and parasitic worms that can enter the body via your feet.

'So no bare feet!' he warned. 'This used to be called the white man's grave. The first people to visit here died.'

I had no intention of having my trip, or my life, cut short by Liberian leeches and worms. I made a mental note to always wear shoes and to take my anti-malarial tablets.

For mile after mile all we could see was the immense green fabric of the forest canopy, until a burnt orange and green patch of land came into view. It turned out to be the landing strip.

Stepping off the plane in the heart of the bush was the moment that I fell in love with Africa. It looked beautiful, with a wonderful aroma. I was dazzled by the bursts of green, red and blue, and the heady scent of flowers and trees in the tropical heat.

The waiting Toyota 4x4 jolted us around the pot-holes along a logging road through the forest. The air was thick with clouds thrown up from the rust-coloured track. The millions of tiny specks were all-pervading, tinting everything like a sepia photograph.

'Everyone here is excited,' Lavoisier said as we stepped out of the truck. 'They look forward to meeting you – their new boss. These are the workers' quarters.'

'Presumptuous with their ambitions for future employment,' I whispered to myself.

I grimaced as I scanned a pathetic selection of run-down wooden huts, with obligatory tin roofs. I found it hard to believe that anyone lived in the most basic of accommodation. In Europe, I murmured to myself, even the cows would turn up their noses.

The men gathered around me in an eager throng while the women and children kept their distance, although they studied me intently. Lavoisier introduced me to everyone in his usual gentle way, and I was given a warm welcome by them all.

Greetings over, and surrounded by emaciated goats and scrawny chickens, we crossed the road to the sawmill. Was this a lame duck? The sawmill appeared to be abandoned, with broken and rusty equipment scattered everywhere around the enormous ten-acre site. The roof, broken and full of holes, sat precariously on top of the flimsy walls.

I pondered over the building's future as I stood surrounded by ancient engines, motor parts, windscreens, propellers and tyres. Undeterred, the ageing generator chugged on and I had to admire its resilience. Most of the buildings were boarded up and, though a few men still worked there, the sawmill had the air of a long-forgotten scrapyard. Thinking back, the forlorn place resembled a graveyard for retired metal parts of any description.

Piles of logs lay around, dumped in disorderly fashion, and the sight of those raw ingredients did give me some hope.

However, there was no feeling of love anywhere, as if no one cared about the site, the building, the equipment or the people who worked there.

A plume of dust hovered around the decaying scene. Time had stood still, with only the generator plodding on towards an uncertain future. I could see that investment was needed; £1 million to get the operation up and running properly, plus a large helping of love and passion.

The wooden, slatted gate creaked and groaned as it closed behind us. We drove on for another thirty minutes to an old landing station, where logs were marked and prepared to go to port.

I could hear an astonishing range of noises in the bush. Animals, out of sight, chattered incessantly. Others made screaming noises. There was rustling all around.

Multi-coloured parrots flew past while a rainbow of butterflies rose from the bone-dry earth. Intense greens of all sizes, shapes and descriptions surrounded me. I was dwarfed by a tangle of foliage, reaching high into the sky.

The scent of the spectacular surroundings smothered me with a wonderful sensation. I could smell the earth; I could taste a minty flavour; I was enveloped in a thousand perfumes. This was virgin bush with a feast for all the senses.

And to think that I had become used to the unwelcoming aroma seeping out of Great Yarmouth fish market. As I breathed in the bold, new fragrances, I believed that I had stepped onto another planet.

Logs lay stacked in rows, rotting into the earth. Clearly the wood had not been sprayed regularly, as it should have been.

By then the heat of the day and the dust of the place and noise of the bush were beginning to affect my mood. The venture was dying, and I had serious doubts that I was the person to bring it back to life.

'Next stop, Port Greenville,' Lavoisier announced as we

returned to the airstrip for the flight down to the coast. 'That's where the ships dock.'

We landed at Greenville where a grass strip sat on the top of a hill, a short drive from the harbour. From the Port of Greenville, Cape Palmas' logs went all over the world where they were sold on to timber merchants and furniture factories.

The roads became ever busier and more chaotic and dusty as we neared the port. We encountered a myriad of logging trucks and 4x4 vehicles. Men and machines threw up clouds of red scorched earth with their every movement. Near the port was a cluster of abandoned twenty-foot shipping containers, rusting away – a slight step up from the crumbling huts. It was a depressing sight and I was shocked, but said nothing.

The quay at the harbour was nearly two hundred metres long and everything appeared to be well built because of foreign investment. Down on the dock, the ships were just as chaotic as everything else in the country. Some listed on their sides, while others were totally dead in the water with broken masts and rusting red hulls.

Of course there were logs everywhere, stacked high and mighty. Two large vessels, ready to be loaded, dominated the quay. They looked like modern day pirate tubs with ropes hanging down into the water. Motley crews leered over the side as they attended to a collection of young ladies, who also lived on the boats and provided a variety of services.

For several minutes Lavoisier and I stood quietly watching all the activity. It brought to mind my earliest working days back in Great Yarmouth in 1968; the contrast between the two ports could not have been greater. In the days I worked there, Great Yarmouth was a busy port with quays either side of the River Yare. There was a constant ebb and flow of boats in and out of the harbour – fishing boats, many oil related supply vessels, but it was always well organised in spite of all the activity. Beyond the port, the infrastructure was equally good and well maintained.

The port at Greenville, for all the dirt, noise and chaos, at least had 20th century facilities; however, immediately beyond the harbour, the town seemed almost out of biblical times.

The way the port functioned was also unlike anything I'd ever seen before, with two ways of loading ships. Logs were either loaded by cranes directly into the vessel's hold, or dropped into the water and pushed across the harbour by paid swimmers. They guided the logs towards on-board cranes, which hoisted the cargo on board as quickly as possible. However, the more dense woods that didn't float were loaded from the quay.

Once the vessels were fully loaded, strong chemical 'bombs' were thrown in the cargo holds to stop the endless variety of local insects from eating through the logs. The hatches were closed quickly, the deck cranes pulled back, and the vessel would drop its tie ropes and depart.

But, no matter how haphazardly the port was run, the frenetic activity told me that there was obviously a huge demand. Cape Palmas Logging might have ground to a halt, but the potential for a bright future appeared to be enormous.

When we landed back at Spriggs Payne Airport late that afternoon our plane interrupted another game of football being played on the runway. It kicked off again after our landing.

That night I struggled to sleep. The country was a complicated one – in fact far more complex than I realised at the time. It was fuelled by forces that I'd yet to see, such as fear and corruption; but all I could envisage was an opportunity to turn a business around and potentially make a decent profit.

When I eventually fell asleep, I dreamed about rebuilding Cape Palmas Logging. At my disposal I had a decrepit sawmill, an endless supply of timber and a willing workforce.

I decided that, if I didn't go ahead, I would only live to

regret missing such an opportunity. One of the smallest African countries, tucked under Sierra Leone, promised me everything. Now was the time for Liberia to match my enthusiasm. However, I realised that the venture would only work with a 'hands-on' approach.

Lavoisier and I spent the next few days meeting an endless stream of dignitaries and suppliers – all eager to have our business. Lavoisier was keen for us to move forward with the deal.

'We need to get going before the rainy season,' he warned.

I, too, was keen to get going. But first I had to sort out mountains of paperwork, agree a contract and get it signed.

Liberia was about to welcome a new resident who was enthralled by the country, its forests – and stunning wildlife.

I fell in love with Africa.

CHAPTER EIGHT

The Mongoose and the Monkey

Chemotherapy continues at St George's Hospital.

Eating has become something of a struggle as the chemotherapy is beginning to make me feel nauseous, although I haven't yet been physically sick. I manage some cereal, toast and a banana, and then take my pills. In addition to my regular small cupful of drugs, I'm now having intravenous anti-sickness medication, topped-up by pills if necessary. Every four hours my blood pressure, pulse and temperature are taken. The Heparin, which prevents blood clots, is constantly administered via a drip and replaced whenever required.

I receive just 50 mg of the chemotherapy drug Fludarabine today, in a saline solution, through the Hickman Line.

Fighting both fatigue and nausea I begin reading the book Vicky bought me, Peterhead Porridge, about life in Scotland's most notorious jail. The other books gifted to me are also about people who spent time in various prisons, and I wonder whether friends and family conferred on the theme of confinement!

My thoughts turn to Axel and what he's going through, all so selflessly, and I feel humbled yet again. Today he begins having Granulocyte injected twice daily to release the stem cells from his bone marrow into his blood stream. He will have these injections for five days prior to travelling four hundred miles to a hospital in Dresden where stem cells will be harvested from his blood.

I am one of around two thousand people in the UK who need a stem cell transplant each year. Of those, around 60%

of haematopoietic stem cell donations are autologous – using the patient's own stem cells. The other 40% are allogeneic – from another person. Thirty per cent of these allogeneic donations are from a related donor, generally a sibling, while 70% are from an unrelated donor or cord blood. [7]

In 2013, three hundred and sixty-seven UK patients received donations from unrelated UK donors, and five hundred and fifty from non-UK based unrelated donors. Every day, as a result of Anthony Nolan's work, three people donate their stem cells to a complete stranger in a selfless attempt to save a life.

After my first transplant, in 2004, I had to wait two years to discover the identity of my donor. Now Axel is part of my family. He has given me life, twice now, and he has pledged to be there for me if needed at any time in the future.

His maturity and generosity inspired me from the start. I was so impressed that a twenty-year old – as he was at the time of my first transplant – would even think about giving a blood sample to be included on a donor register.

In the afternoon my brother Gary brings me a more comfortable pillow and a table to complete a jigsaw puzzle. The puzzle has been made especially for me and features my granddaughters and their dog, Skye. It is a gift from Louisa.

After Gary's visit I pass the time listening to music, watching movement in the corridor outside and some TV. I'm so thankful that I have this room giving me a view, and also for the exemplary 24-hour care of the staff. It is my aim to be the least needy of their patients, and I've set myself the challenge of not using the call button at all during my stay. A nurse reminds me that I do need monitoring! I did at least last a week before my telling off.

---

7   Cord blood is the blood that remains in the placenta and umbilical cord after a baby is born. Usually, after birth, the placenta and umbilical cord are thrown away; however, as this is a rich source of stem cells, the NHS Cord Blood Bank was set up in 1996 to collect, process, store and supply cord blood for transplants.

Come the evening, I Face Time Vicky, Louisa and my brother David, and it's good to have the outside world brought to me through them; but aside from that I'm feeling exhausted and happy. It's time to take a pill and escape into sleep, dreaming about a monkey and a mongoose...

★★★

I imagined that signing the contract with Cape Palmas Logging would be straightforward. Here I was, in a struggling African country, offering to invest and turn a business around. I was about to offer employment and make a contribution to the local economy. I thought that all of this would make the signing a simple process. Wrong.

Enter Esther, Lavoisier's wife. Unbelievably, she had been trying to negotiate a separate deal for the company behind all of our backs. However, she did not succeed and finally, in September 1988, I flew back to Liberia to sign the agreement with Lavoisier. From that point onwards, Lavoisier kept his wife well away from the business and me.

I now owned 51% of Cape Palmas Logging, with 374,000 acres of trees under licence from the Forestry Development Authority of Liberia.[8] The licence had an annual fee of $180,000, a large percentage of which was to pay for extensive reforestation programmes within the country. We were finally ready to go; except that the rainy season had by then begun, turning the roads into thick mud, allowing few vehicles to pass. Until that time, no logging could begin.

There was still so much to be done: hire new staff where needed; meet with the Forest Development Authority; assess and pay valid creditors; order necessary plant, machinery and vehicles; and visit appropriate government agencies among

---

8   Liberia has 160 inches of rain every year, or more than thirteen feet

endless other tasks. Firstly, I wanted to fly back to the sawmill and Cape Palmas' tracts of forest in Sinoe County.

We were trying to revive a business in the middle of nowhere with no running water, electricity or basic essentials.

Once more we flew over the rainforest in one of Quinca's tiny planes, but this time it was the rainy season. Thick clouds of steam hung over the trees and dark tentacles of water coursed amongst them.

Lavoisier pointed out where river banks had burst and bridges had broken or been swept away. It was clear to see why the logging business ground to a halt during the rainy season.

When we entered the Cape Palmas compound, I was astonished to see every man, woman and child connected to the company waiting to give us an enthusiastic welcome. Once again there were endless hands to shake. Over and over the people told me how grateful they were that I had saved the company – and their livelihoods.

'Bossman,' someone called, and soon the crowd had taken up the chant. 'Bossman! Welcome Bossman! Bossman!' I waved, embarrassed at all the attention, but also pleased that I was making a difference to their lives.

We were escorted to the main house on the compound, where the cook had miraculously prepared bacon and eggs and sweet tea for Lavoisier and me.

There was a knock at the door and three of the elders, dressed in threadbare western business suits, were waiting to formally meet Bossman. One of the elders carried a thin chicken while another of them was leading a scrawny white goat, both of which were handed ceremoniously to me as gifts from the people. I made a short speech, expressing my thanks. I was slightly alarmed when the cook grabbed the animals and, despite their obvious displeasure, bolted off in the direction of the kitchen.

We continued exchanging pleasantries, and the company's future, while a succession of squawks and shrieks came from the kitchen.

'Welcome to the Jungle' by Guns N' Roses was a hit at the time and the words filled my head. Instead a rough sounding cassette player did its best to play 'Hungry Eyes' by Eric Carmen, another big seller from the period.

I lost my appetite completely when the cook reappeared, having silenced the larger of the two protesting victims with his finely-honed kitchen accessories. As if taking part in a ceremony, he carried a large tureen into the lounge. He placed it before me and revealed the poor goat's balls presented on a skewer.

'Eat!' the elders urged, all smiles.

But I was truly ready to be sick and, much as I knew I was causing offence, there was no way that I could consume the offering. Somehow the chicken found a reprieve from its death sentence that day; probably because there was no meat on the creature to eat.

One of my tasks on that trip was to assess the need for new machinery. The list was long – and eye-wateringly expensive. When the first order was finally placed, we spent a staggering US$1,000,000 on essential equipment. That included a Caterpillar D7G to plough our way into the jungle, a road grader to construct a flat surface for vehicles, and two Caterpillar Skidders to pull out the logs.

We also ordered reconditioned trucks, a Caterpillar 966 and logging trailers from Belgium. From England, we acquired a new water tank and trucks at a British Army sale. These had to be painted white for the sea voyage, so that the Liberians didn't think they were being invaded! We also bought new chainsaws and vital communications equipment for the bush. In addition, I bought a used Range Rover to use in Monrovia and two Safari Land Rovers[9] to tackle the formidable terrain.

Since there was no infrastructure in the bush, everything had to be brought in ourselves: food, petrol for the machines and generators, spare tyres for the Caterpillar vehicles (these regularly split or broke and cost an astonishing $5,000 each), and endless other essentials. It was a two-day trip just to get there by road – when the going was good. Nevertheless, within a few days, everything that I'd bought in Monrovia set off in a long and dusty convoy for our bush camp in Sinoe County. The vehicles and other equipment, expected from Europe, would take around two to three months to arrive.

By then I'd also rented a sizable house with an office in Sinkor, the same district where Lavoisier lived. It appeared to be lavish – a familiar story in the country – although on closer inspection a lot of things didn't work. Nevertheless, it was where Siafa Sherman, our office manager, would be based. The house also had a small room at the back, which was ideal for our radio equipment – necessary for keeping in touch with activities in the bush, as well as the port and sawmill.

A veranda and colourful garden attracted a kaleidoscope of local songbirds; a welcome oasis and an escape from the chaos of the city. Siafa was a well-educated, astute and gentle man who had worked for Lavoisier for a number of years and was certainly an asset to the company. We also hired a cook, a housekeeper and a gatekeeper. I bought a dog to keep rats and other unwelcome pests at bay.

Other staff were needed to build up the Cape Palmas team. I hired a Spanish man, Antonio Vasquez, who was an experienced bushman. He acted as bush manager, organising the transport of supplies and equipment from Monrovia to Sinoe, and logs from Sinoe to the Port of Greenville – a round

---

9   This version of the Land Rover has a second roof skin with vents fitted on top of the vehicle to keep the interior cool in hot weather, and reduce condensation when it's cooler.

trip of three hundred miles. He was a key man when it came to plan each day's felling.

We were also joined by Herbert, a German engineer and sawmill operator, who had lived and worked in Africa for a while. He was a small mountain of muscle and started work immediately. Before long he had brought much of the machinery back to life. This included the all-important sawmill and welding shop. He then turned his attention to the logs in the yard. I spent a lot of time in the sawmill, simply watching the wood being sliced into timber. Observing the huge machines was mesmerising; the smell of the freshly-sawn wood had a distinct and wonderful aroma.

Herbert then set about salvaging logs that had lain abandoned for two years – as much as they could be, given the weather and plethora of insects. He seemed to relish working eighteen hour days and, within a couple of weeks, he'd revitalised and organised the whole place. Finally, the new vehicles arrived from Britain, though they took an age – and some sizable backhanders – to clear customs. They certainly attracted plenty of attention as we drove them in convoy from the port to the Cape Palmas base, horns honking and red dust rising all the way. Cape Palmas Logging was back in business.

Before long Antonio Vasquez had discovered a valuable source of timber on the other side of a fast-flowing river on our land. I watched intently as a group of workers created a road down to the river. Then, using ironwood cut in our sawmill, they constructed a bridge in less than three days. While it was certainly rudimentary in design and form, it was able to cope with hundreds of tons of vehicles, equipment and logs.

Once we reached the bank on the other side of the river, the land was so densely packed with vegetation that you could barely see more than a metre ahead. Sometimes I'd catch the outline of a monkey high in the forest canopy or see a parrot briefly through the foliage. But while the many and varied inhabitants remained mostly hidden, you could certainly hear a great number of them. Hundreds of birds screeched and twittered, while wild boars padded through the undergrowth. The noise was unquestionably charming during the daytime; however at night, with the volume turned up, it could be truly terrifying.

Our next task after building the bridge was to construct a road deeper into the forest and prepare a clearing for a landing station. This was where the trees, bare of branches, were brought out from the bush and graded into logs for exporting. These were measured and marked for identification before being taken to Port Greenville for shipping. Once the landing station was up and running, I hired a night watchman to guard both the equipment and logs kept overnight at the site. He was unusually lanky for a Liberian and had a calm and quiet manner that lent itself well to his job. I had heard that he was a bushman through and through, but was still a little surprised when he turned up with a rifle for his first night's work.

The following morning at sun-up, when Antonio and I returned to the landing station, I was horrified to see the night watchman sitting on a log. He was calmly smoking a cigarette, with a pile of chewed bones and a small broken skull by his feet. Had he consumed a child? Antonio, sensing my shock, laughed and by way of explanation said, 'Monkey!' Once again I realised how out of step I was with local eating habits. The monkey's brains were an early morning delicacy for the bushman.

Another day in the bush, the truck drivers combined to prepare a rare delicacy. They boiled water in a bucket, tied over a fire and shone a torch into the water. I had no idea what to expect, but soon white-bodied moths with transparent wings followed the light into the bucket. I felt uncomfortable watching the process.

'How many do you need?' I asked.

'Just watch!' they said. Soon, literally hundreds of these insects were drawn to the light and quickly stirred into the water. The bush workers considered this a special event and meal, though I declined to taste the soup.

One morning we arrived at the landing station, where the logs were stored, awaiting shipment to Port Greenville.

We were all ready to start work when a mechanic came over to me and said that the Caterpillar D7G would not start. I asked what the problem was.

He said the starter motor appeared to be missing.

'So where are we going to get one in the middle of the bush?' I asked tetchily.

'I know a friend who has a starter motor for the Caterpillar.'

'How long will it take to get it? And how much?'

'About twenty minutes,' my nervous mechanic replied. 'Ten dollars.'

I knew what he was up to. I produced the ten Liberian dollars, equivalent to US$4 at the time.

'If this ever happens again I'll call the police. Understand?'

Miraculously, the starter motor reappeared and was fitted to the vehicle. There was no repeat incident.

As the business quickly re-established itself, the weather grew increasingly hot and humid. The weather was only bearable in the mornings, with fresh breezes coming in off the Atlantic. As soon as the sun came up, the weight of humidity weighed us all down. The dense forest vegetation gave respite from direct sunlight, but it was still stiflingly hot with insects scuttling, creeping or flying at every turn. Many were six and even seven inches in length.

Our concession of land, 374,000 acres of this forest, was for our use only. It was separated from our neighbours by 'the line'. This area had to be kept clear of any vegetation, with no unexpected visitors. In Liberia possession is one hundred per cent of the law, so anyone could theoretically enter your land and steal your logs.

Therefore, from time to time, our ranger would 'walk the line' to check that all was as it should be. I realised that, to earn his respect, I would have to walk it with him one day.

'Bossman, this will be very difficult for you,' he warned me. 'We will walk from six in the morning to six at night, in the heat, over rivers and through swamps with mosquitoes.'

I had committed myself to doing it and would not back out. We set off early in the morning, when the bush was arguably at its most beautiful. Vivid parrots patrolled the trees and accompanied us as we walked; red ants marched purposefully across our path; and the light on the leaves and smell of it all was wonderful. However, I had to be wary of dangerous roots, or narrow paths, especially when the canopy thickened and shut out much of the light.

By the end of that day, I was exhausted and aching all over when we arrived at the ranger's tin-roofed hut in the midst of the jungle. His wife welcomed us with a smile and a bucket each of hot water, for us to shower with. I was given food and a beautifully made bed. I suspect that they had borrowed the linen especially for me, as it was so out of place with everything else. The only drawback was a persistent swarm of cockroaches, determined to share my bed. I barely slept a moment, though of course I said nothing to the ranger or his wife.

Before long, with the business gathering momentum, we reopened the office in Port Greenville. There was also a company-owned house with a resident mongoose to keep snakes, rats and mice at bay. Whenever I needed to go to Greenville, I would charter one of Quinca's planes and the pilot would buzz the office to let them know we were landing.

We also had a yard close to the port, where we stored our logs for buyers to inspect our stock and await shipment.

The yard was large and boggy at one end, probably with sea water as it was very close to the ocean. One day I walked down to the far end of the yard where our logs awaited shipment. I stood there. pleased with the load we had accumulated. I glanced over to my right and, not ten feet away, was an equally long crocodile! My immediate thought was not to panic, though my body had other ideas and I instinctively leaped several feet up onto a log. As I found my footing, I looked down at the crocodile's bulging eyes. I flinched. The croc's eyes bulged even more. He swished his tail and continued to eye me up. I was definitely on his dinner menu. Using every ounce of strength in my body, I clambered up over the pile of logs and beat the hastiest of retreats.

I loved the sights and sounds of Greenville port. I'd always enjoyed the atmosphere at Great Yarmouth and Aberdeen ports, despite the vastly different surroundings. Loading was especially fascinating, although I learned how dangerous the work of 'swimming' the logs to a ship could be. The bobbing logs and water movement posed lethal hazards to these brave 'swimmers'. Just imagine diving under a huge log with a rope, securing the rope to a hook, and guiding the massive piece of timber alongside a waiting ship – with cranes hovering, ready to claim their cargo. Health and Safety would have had a field day.

I also enjoyed spending my evenings in the bars along the port, listening to tales from the sailors of every nationality who convened there. Occasionally, I was an invited guest on the international vessels in port who offered the best food and beer in town to their customers. Of course, I was always happy to be on the receiving end of their generous hospitality.

In Monrovia the street cafes and bars were also interesting places to visit. They were far from chic; in fact it was not uncommon for rats to scuttle between the grubby formica tables and rickety chairs. One day I had popped into a cafe to grab a morning coffee between meetings, when I suddenly felt as though I'd been cudgelled over the head. The pain was so intense that I could barely move – even finishing my coffee was impossible. I managed to get my driver's attention. He scooped me into the Range Rover and sped back to the house.

Once there, Siafa put his hand to my forehead and said simply, 'Malaria'. Having consistently taken my anti-malarial tablets each week, the diagnosis was particularly annoying; but this was obviously some exceptionally virulent strain. I was put to bed immediately, and before long I was unable to even lift my head from the pillow. Sweat coursed off my body, and for the next five days, the pain was so excruciating that even going to the toilet – a regular feature of the illness – was a major ordeal. I certainly couldn't eat, barely slept, and felt as if I'd lost all control of my body. I grew weaker by the day, to the point where it was a struggle to grip a glass or even to stand. I lost ten pounds in weight in half as many days.

My recovery was slow, haphazard, and painful. The fever would recede and then come back again and hit me like a tsunami. To begin with I could only tolerate the noise of the mynah birds in the garden, but after a while I was able to add the crackle of the radio to keep me company. Siafa became a bulwark between the business and me, quietly and calmly taking care of whatever needed attending to. An English woman called Jane, who worked in a restaurant close by, surprised me by providing a complimentary bowl of spiced chicken soup for lunch every day. Little by little I gained my strength until I was finally able to walk again; and, as my health returned, my friendship grew with Jane.

Before my illness, she'd come across as distant and cold. However, her daily acts of kindness showed that was not the case at all. It was a real lesson for me, giving someone a second chance after a bad first impression.

With Cape Palmas going from strength to strength, and

having regained my own, I began to realise that back in Jersey Sue was feeling somewhat neglected, so I invited her over for a visit – after which she decided to stay. Sue took to life in Liberia immediately, and I was delighted to have her there.

She adored both life in Monrovia and the raw beauty of the bush, which she was confident in exploring on her own. She also loved Port Greenville with its frenetic activity and weekday market. The air was always fragrant with coconuts and yams, papayas and plantain, and endless other foods that I never learned to name.

Sue had a great way, not only with people, but also with animals: from our dog Buster in Monrovia to the chickens we kept. She was also fond of all the wild animals and birds. Her reputation with animals was such that one day, when Sue was staying behind in the staff house as I headed into the bush, I asked her to look after a young chimpanzee belonging to Antonio, the bush manager.

Antonio had assured us that the chimpanzee was quite tame; however, Sue's inner Dr. Doolittle had finally met its nemesis. The young chimp was impervious to her charms. It spent hours seemingly determined to torment her – pulling at her hair, screaming its annoyance, and literally climbing the walls. Eventually, Sue had had enough of the furry toddler's tantrums and locked the chimp in a small room off the kitchen.

Calm reigned once again in the house and Sue relaxed into a book. Suddenly, the peace of the afternoon was shattered by the sound of smashing glass. Sue edged anxiously in the direction of the small room beside the kitchen, from where the sound had emerged. Tentatively, she unlocked the door and was surprised when the chimp didn't immediately make a bid for freedom. She was aware of a pungent smell as she turned on the light; the pong turned out to be alcohol and chimpanzee pooh. And in the corner, clutching a bottle of bush whisky in its hand, was the drunken culprit. Sue cleaned up the chimp and nursed him through his hangover until Antonio came home that evening, but kept her distance after that.

Sue was probably not thrilled when, shortly after that, I brought home a small monkey with an orange ruff around its black triangular face. The animal was a gift from a local shopkeeper. She reluctantly accepted the animal and I set off back into the bush.

I returned at lunchtime to a cacophony of screams. They were so loud that I feared for Sue's life. I dashed into the lounge and saw that Sue was being terrorised by the monkey. The berserk creature was shrieking at Sue while trying to latch on to her breast. I ran off in search of the house mongoose, in the hope that it might come to the rescue.

'No, don't do that,' insisted Sue. 'The cook put him in the back room. The animals don't get on.'

'They'll be fine!' I assured her,

However, I should have listened to the cook. The mongoose bolted from the room and raced to the monkey, screeching its fury at the sight of an enemy. Seeking refuge, the monkey leaped on my head, with its vicious claws digging into my scalp. From then on the two of them had to be separated at all times. Eventually, when I grew tired of all the squabbling, I returned the monkey to the shopkeeper.

'Do you have a problem?' the shopkeeper asked, frowning at the monkey.

'Yes, the arrangement hasn't quite worked out.'

'I am sure you can get on. It just takes time to build a relationship.'

'No, no,' I explained. 'Your monkey has taking a liking to my girlfriend. On top of that, there is a mongoose in the house.'

'You've got a mongoose?' he gasped. 'You must know all about a mongoose and a monkey?'

'That is the problem. Sue and your monkey have spats. The mongoose will ensure a fight to the death.'

One nil to the mongoose.

Shortly afterwards, Sue noticed that the skin on her ankle was swelling and turning red.

Thinking it was a mosquito bite she ignored it but gradually, as it numbed, Sue's anxiety grew. She stood up and felt dizzy, so decided to go downstairs and ask Siafa for his opinion.

'Madame, we need to take you to hospital immediately,' he urged, after inspecting the wound. 'Spider bite, Madame.'

Sue quickly grabbed her bag and then Siafa sped off in one of the company trucks, over the potholes and through the traffic to a ramshackle open-air building. When they arrived, Sue thought he'd made a mistake.

'No Madame, this is the hospital,' he insisted, leading her towards one of the nurses on duty.

Within moments, she was put on her back, her leg raised in a noose, and given a huge shot of antibiotics. The hospital staff thought that she'd probably be all right, but that she'd have to keep her leg raised as high as possible for two days. When the bandages were removed a couple of days later, there were two dark and distinct fang marks in her skin. I would have quite understood if, at that stage Sue had demanded to return home to Europe. However, she bravely decided to stay.

I'd been more concerned with Sue's brush with the spider and death than I let on; mostly because Liberian hospitals had such a bad reputation for doing more harm than good. Fortunately, Sue had come through the incident and made a full recovery.

All the logging companies paid health insurance for their expatriate employees. Medical evacuations, by jet to Europe, were a common occurrence.

I learned this early on during my stay in Liberia, when

I was introduced to an affable Englishman called Bill who worked for another logging company. He was tall with blond hair and striking blue eyes. Over a few beers he told me about the inside workings of the industry – the greasing of palms, the Machiavellian manoeuvring of the FDA, and the endless negotiating all around. He enthused about seeing his wife and new baby back in Yorkshire over Christmas. When I left for my hotel, we parted and agreed to meet again sometime soon.

It was not to be. Tragically, later that night, he was travelling in a car which crashed into a parked logging truck in the pitch dark. One of the logs decapitated him in an instant. Remarkably, the driver walked away uninjured, but another passenger sustained multiple injuries and was medically evacuated back to the UK for treatment.

Unfortunately accidents like these were all too commonplace in Liberia; with the badly maintained narrow roads and appalling standard of driving, it was probably no real surprise. What was slightly surprising was the off-hand reaction from many of the old-hand ex-pats, who seemed almost unmoved by such events. In fact, all around there was an apparent acceptance of circumstances that would have been completely unacceptable in Europe.

Bribery was one such thing. During the two years that I lived in Liberia, I paid vast amounts of money – tens of thousands of dollars – to a high ranking official with the FDA. This ensured that the paperwork for my logs passed through the ridiculous – and corrupt – red-tape labyrinth.

All too often, while I enjoyed watching logs being lowered into a vessel at Port Greenville, a call came through from my FDA nemesis. He demanded that shipment should be halted and that I should visit his office, one hundred and fifty miles away in Monrovia.

On several occasions I had to charter a plane from Quinca and fly up to Monrovia and then be kept waiting in his office for hours at a time. It was all part of his manipulative tactics to escalate the tension.

After one of these hold-ups, costing me a lot of time and money, I was making my way back to the office when my driver suggested that we both pop into a shack en-route for a bite to eat.

'Bossman, only be ten minutes,' he said.

Only I just didn't have the time, as I knew from experience that a 'quick lunch' in Monrovia inevitably stretched into an hour at the very least, and I had to get supplies for the bush and catch a plane. So I let him go in for lunch – giving him the money to take a bus back home – and drove the Range Rover back to the office myself. There, much to my surprise, I was greeted by a furious Siafa.

'Eric,' he said, 'do you have any idea how dangerous it is for a man like you to drive alone? You're an easy target.'

He was right. Civil unrest was escalating. Murders were becoming commonplace. I'd become so caught up in rebuilding Cape Palmas Logging that I hadn't taken full account of the changing political landscape.

I had become too concerned with my own grand adventure. I was consumed by ambitions in the bush.

Samuel Doe's grasp on affairs – never that firm – was slipping, and the country simmered with discontent.

Liberia was on the brink of a precipice. Uncertainty fuelled fear. I could smell and taste that fear.

A feeling of hopelessness enveloped the entire country.

CHAPTER NINE

Children in the Bush

July 27th 2014. Day five at St George's Hospital, London.

Again, I'm feeling quite sick, but nevertheless eat a small amount of cereal, toast and a banana. The routine of pills and monitoring from the staff is very familiar now, as is the dose of chemotherapy – the same type and quantity as yesterday – and I submit to the rhythm of it all.

More than anything, I'm feeling tired and even reading or attempting my puzzle is a struggle. Thinking does not require much energy, and I turn my thoughts to my family, what they mean to me, and my hopes for the future. Work seems so much less important now, and what I would like is to be in a position of freedom; to visit my family at any time.

Gary comes back again in the afternoon, but apart from that I try to rest as much as possible between the regular visits from hospital staff, attempts at eating, and a few Face Time calls from my family. I can't thank Gary enough for his constant care and support.

I'm pleased when it's late enough to take a sleeping pill and retreat from the day into sleep.

July 28th 2014. Day six at St George's Hospital, London.

In the morning I make a stab at breakfast, not because I'm hungry, but because my weight has dropped by two kilos since my admission. However, the staff do their utmost to mitigate the nausea with medication, and I'm reminded of my good fortune in having their attention. Also, there has been a marked improvement in anti-sickness medication since my last transplant ten years ago, so I'm grateful for that too.

Today I'm administered a test dose of a special drug, Anti-Thymocyte Globulin (ATG), a rabbit-derived serum that – it is hoped – will prevent my body rejecting my donor's stem cells and also prevent the donor cells from attacking me later on; a condition called graft versus host disease. Some people react badly to this drug, which is why I'm being given the test dose.

I develop a severe headache after the ATG and take the day slowly to let my body have the rest it clearly craves. Hospital staff deliver sandwiches, cereal and rice pudding, plus the obligatory medicine. I Face Time my family in the evening. However, when the time comes for me to take my sleeping pill for the night, I feel somewhat relieved.

July 29th 2014. Day seven at St George's Hospital, London.

The next morning begins with the familiar routine of health monitoring and attempts to eat cereal and toast, and at 9 a.m. I'm given 60mg of Methylprednisolene, 10mg of Chlorphenimine, and then at noon I begin receiving 162.5mg of ATG in 500mls of saline solution. These take twelve hours to drip into my body.

Two hours into the procedure, I start to feel worsening pain in my lower legs. Before long, I'm feeling constantly nauseous and have a chronic headache and high temperature, for which I'm given codeine and paracetamol.

These ease the pain, though it continues for the remaining ten hours of the ATG infusion. During all this time I can barely eat or sleep, and I'm certainly not up to making Face Time calls, even to my daughters. It takes all my strength of mind to visualise myself through this process, becoming well again, and not dwelling on the pain. I am tempted to receive a boost from my favourite songs, but decide that I can hold on for

the time being. I'm relieved when the day finally passes and I reflect on
some of my bizarre dealings in Africa…

★★★

I woke up to the reality that Liberia was becoming a dangerous place for both locals and expatriates alike. I had my ear to the ground to keep tabs on the country's troubles, while I pushed on with the business.

You could never be too sure of what you were being told. Just like any town or city in any country, Monrovia's bars were hotspots for gossip and rumours. I enjoyed listening to cracking tales about other companies, dodgy deals or bizarre transactions. I took it all with a rather large pinch of salt.

Monrovia is the political, financial and cultural hub of Liberia. All the government offices, including the FDA, with whom I had regular dealings, were in the town as were many of our suppliers such as Caterpillar where we bought machinery and tyres. There were also dozens of smaller but nevertheless essential businesses. Everything that was imported into Liberia – from containers of cigarettes or rice, pig trotters in brine, alcohol or chicken feet – came through Monrovia.

Trade was the lifeblood of much of Liberia, and talk often fuelled that trade, so I always kept an ear out for interesting snippets. I usually drank in a hotel bar off Benson Street, one of the main thoroughfares in Monrovia, where locals and expats mingled and traded tall stories. On one occasion, I entered a conversation about diamonds and talk of a trader who owned a bush cafe and store. He was dealing with a few diamonds each week, brought to him by children. I loved the story, although it was hard to believe.

During my time in Liberia I had often heard of people profiting from diamonds and gold. However, there was something about this piece of gossip that intrigued me – I felt compelled to investigate further.

Discreetly, I tried to find out more: mainly, the bush café's location. Many conversations later, I had a rough idea that I would be looking for a tiny settlement fifty to sixty miles outside of Monrovia, on the main road heading east into the bush.

After my bout of malaria I decided to take things easier and have some time to myself. The following Sunday – a month or so after first hearing about the unlikely trade – I decided to take a rare day off from my business. I was eager to find this rumoured bush cafe where children brought diamonds to sell.

I loaded ten 28-lb bags of rice into the Range Rover – just in case I hit the jackpot – and, with my driver Jerome, set off with a tank full of petrol to the eastern outskirts of the city. Rice is a staple food in Liberia, although too expensive for many families to buy regularly, so I knew it would be a prized offering.

As we drove off I wondered: would the journey end up as a wild goose chase? Was the tale actually true? Were there really children in the bush, prepared to trade diamonds for rice?

The city streets were empty that morning. Once outside Monrovia, we picked up speed but the concrete roads soon petered out into the brown, scorched earth of Africa's bush country. We drove amongst the dust bowls and potholes, throwing up plumes of fine soil in a trail behind us, even though this was a major road used – and maintained – by the logging companies. I kept an eye on the milometer, and once we were around forty miles from the city, we slowed so that I could pay full attention to any tracks or side roads. After fifty miles there was still no sign of a trading post or bush cafe and, slightly disappointed, we carried on.

Finally, up ahead, about eighty-five miles out of Monrovia,

we came to a junction on a bend, leading to the right. Even though it was a Sunday, there were people hanging around or sitting beside the road selling brightly coloured fruit and vegetables. Naturally we slowed down and, on the side road off to the left, I spotted a building. I felt the hairs rise on my neck and a shiver run down my spine. We turned into the road and I asked Jerome to pull up and stop immediately opposite the building.

These trading posts were always built at junctions where locals had traditionally come out from the bush to sell their goods and socialise. This one was a typical trader's business: a concrete house with living quarters upstairs, a shop and cafe downstairs, and a fenced-in compound at the back housing the car and various outbuildings. A high fence was topped with barbed wire, and a loud dog patrolled the premises. A generator hummed away. This was like a small fortress in the bush.

As I stepped down from the Range Rover, all heads turned my way. I was dressed quite casually in jeans, an off-white shirt and brown boots; nevertheless a white man with a black driver stopping at a bush cafe was not a regular occurrence. Just like anywhere else in Liberia, from the airport to the city, to a local it represented a potential trading opportunity.

But on this occasion, it was probably me who was the most excited at the possible prospect of doing a trade. However, I restrained my enthusiasm as I walked across to the building. The place was fully open with the shutters rolled up. At the front was a patio with a wooden floor and a few tables and chairs scattered across it. Behind, stretched a counter and stools where people could pass the time over a Coke or coffee.

Further into the trading post it was an Aladdin's Cave. From top to bottom and left to right the shelves were brimming with tins and jars of food, brooms, brushes and bins, bags of sugar and tea. On the floor, between sleeping stray cats and dogs, were large sacks of rice.

'Let me get you a coffee, you must be thirsty today!' called out the proprietor as he beckoned me over.

He was short, stout and hairy. His wife – the same shape and size – soon appeared by his side followed by two brightly dressed small children.

I guessed they were a Lebanese family, since the majority of shops were owned by Lebanese people who also dominated the currency market. They made vast amounts trading Liberian and US dollars. Officially the currency was set at one Liberian dollar to the US dollar; however, if you were not Lebanese they set it nearer five to one.

I sat and had a drink with the owner, who was clearly curious about my visit to his store. We spoke about everything except diamonds and he asked every permutation of who, what, where, when and how, to try to work out my agenda. He obviously knew that a white man appearing in a Range Rover had funds, and he was also desperate to sell me something. For my part I was wondering whether I was in the right place, or whether this was just another watering hole on yet another logging route.

I decided to broach the subject by asking whether there was any prospecting for gold going on in the area, and he answered 'yes', but that was much further inland. He appeared disinterested in the subject, so I thought I'd push it further.

'Any diamonds?' I added.

'No, only logging,' he said, without the slightest hesitation in his voice. 'Logging trucks pass through here every day.'

It wasn't a route that my own trucks took. But I felt that I was in the wrong place to find the children who traded diamonds – if they existed at all. Perhaps my new friend deserved an Oscar.

We talked some more and I returned to our vehicle. A few people were hanging around and, once again, all eyes were on me. Some children were playing with an old tyre and stick, trying to keep it rolling. I asked my driver to invite them over.

There were several boys and two girls and they ranged from around four to eight years old. Naturally, they appeared to be a little on the shy side.

I wanted to get their attention, so I asked directly: 'I want to buy diamonds. They look like small pieces of glass and have funny shapes.'

I wasn't really expecting any reaction, but then one of them said – in a strange form of broken English – that they'd found similar objects. Another child said the shiny stones weren't hard to find.

Astonished at what I was hearing, I opened the tailgate and showed the children the ten large bags of rice.

'I will give you one sack of rice for any size diamond and I will come back next Sunday to see if you have any.'

These children were fit and lean, and clearly had enough to eat; nevertheless they all understood that a large sack of rice was a valuable commodity to their families and looked at me, amazed at my offer. A large bag or rice cost more than most Liberians earned in a month.

Once my driver had assured them that I was not insane and my offer was genuine, they said they would be back the following Sunday. I asked them to keep it a secret among themselves, which they agreed to; I hardly expected them to keep quiet. I watched the children wander off down the hill and back into the bush. I was thrilled that I'd managed to make my plans, away from the prying eyes and ears of the Lebanese trader.

Although I drove away without a diamond, I was really excited at what I'd set in motion. Three hours later, when I returned to the compound and the gates closed behind me, I remembered what I had thought that morning and reflected: you never know unless you go. I went to bed contemplating what can be achieved if you're prepared to be pro-active and give the long shots a chance. At the time it never occurred to me to question the morality of what I was about to do; however, time and conflict would change all that.

The following week passed quickly. I endured all the usual dramas and problems involved in running a logging company in Liberia. I made two trips down to Port Greenville to negotiate with the port captain. By the end of all that, I was eager to return to Monrovia – straining at the leash for my trip into the bush.

All week, at the back of my mind, I was looking forward to my adventure. I wondered if the children would be there and, if so, would they have the diamonds? One thing was certain: I would have the rice.

Sunday soon came around again. We left at dawn, laden with sacks of rice, and we arrived at the bush cafe by 9.30 a.m. We were a little early, but I had no intention of missing the children. It was still quiet at the trading post with few people about. I strolled over to the cafe and greeted my Lebanese friend.

Within twenty or so minutes the same boys and two girls appeared in the distance. My heart raced as they approached. As they came towards me I stepped away from the cafe, out of hearing distance. We huddled in a circle near the Range Rover and they opened a cloth to reveal four shining diamonds. I was truly astonished. I dropped the tailgate and asked the driver to take out four twenty-eight pound bags of rice. At this point the children gaped in amazement. They were thrilled to take such a valuable commodity back into the bush. To them, it was a fair deal.

Transaction over, I bought them each a cold Coke and they relaxed as trust grew between us. Apart from the drone of the store's generator there was little noise and, when the children had finished their drinks, I told them I'd be back in two weeks with more rice. They were delighted. The boys were almost dwarfed by the bags as they balanced the priceless food on their heads and strolled happily down the hill. I felt both happy and sad as I watched them go, thinking about our totally different worlds. I also thought about my own girls, who were fortunate to be born in luxury, thousands of miles from the poverty of the bush.

We drove back to Monrovia in silence. We said nothing at all for the entire eighty-five miles. My thoughts drifted back to other matters as we returned to familiar landmarks and scenery. Soon enough I was in the home office, with the colourful mynah birds in the tree by the window, next to the radio. They were a calming influence as I had to deal with issue after issue; it was a means of escape for me as nature became more important in my life.

The endless problems of a logging business crackled out of that receiver. The incessant, whining gibberish kept part of my mind occupied – but most of my thoughts were concentrating on trading diamonds for rice.

CHAPTER TEN

Diamonds for Rice

July 30th 2014. Day eight at St George's Hospital, London.

I haven't had a restful night, and I've barely eaten during the last twenty-four hours. Nevertheless, this is quite common during chemotherapy and the staff are unstinting in their care. Thankfully, as the morning progresses, yesterday's pain abates and my appetite returns.

The doctors have advised me that the second day of ATG is often much easier for patients; I'm certainly hoping that's the case as I'm shortly to receive exactly the same drugs and doses as yesterday.

Without question the most noticeable differences between my last transplant and this one, are the advances that have been made in anti-sickness medication. As I sit in my chair having the second large dose of ATG I'm braced for another storm of pain, which happily never comes. Later on I am also given an intravenous infusion of 95mg of Cyclosporine.

Today Axel is at the hospital in Dresden, more than four hundred miles from his village near Munster, having stem cells harvested from his body. Blood is taken by a tube from a vein in one arm, passed into a machine that separates out the stem cells, and then returned into the other arm.

The process will take around four hours, and his blood will be passed through the machine four times to extract as many stem cells as possible. The minimum number required for my donation is two million cells per kilogram of body weight; however, to put this vast quantity into perspective, the human body makes approximately 2.4 million new blood cells every second.

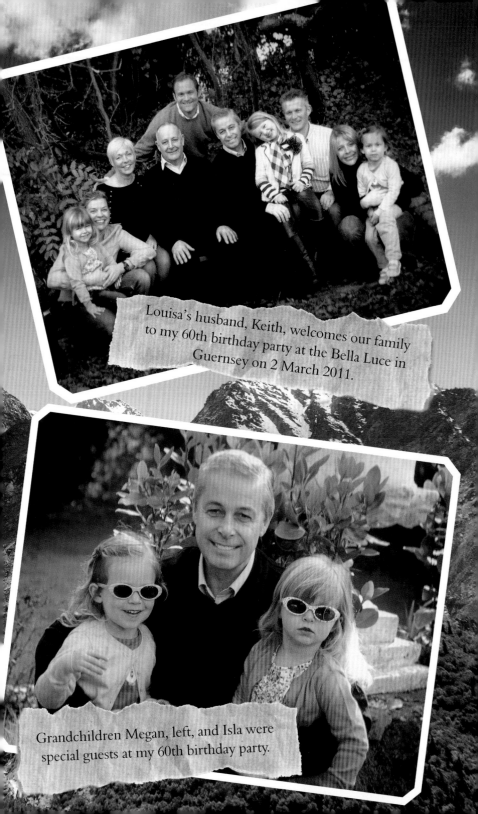

Louisa's husband, Keith, welcomes our family to my 60th birthday party at the Bella Luce in Guernsey on 2 March 2011.

Grandchildren Megan, left, and Isla were special guests at my 60th birthday party.

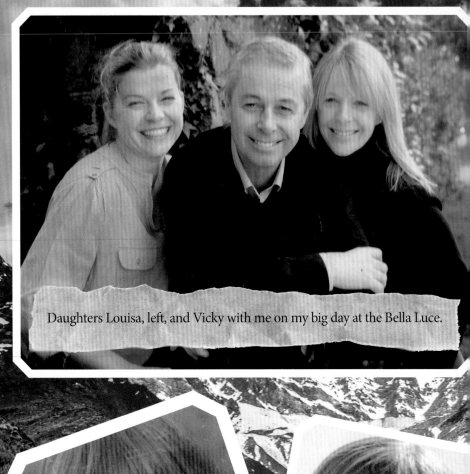

Daughters Louisa, left, and Vicky with me on my big day at the Bella Luce.

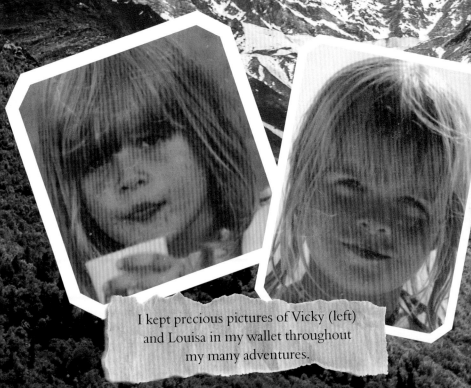

I kept precious pictures of Vicky (left) and Louisa in my wallet throughout my many adventures.

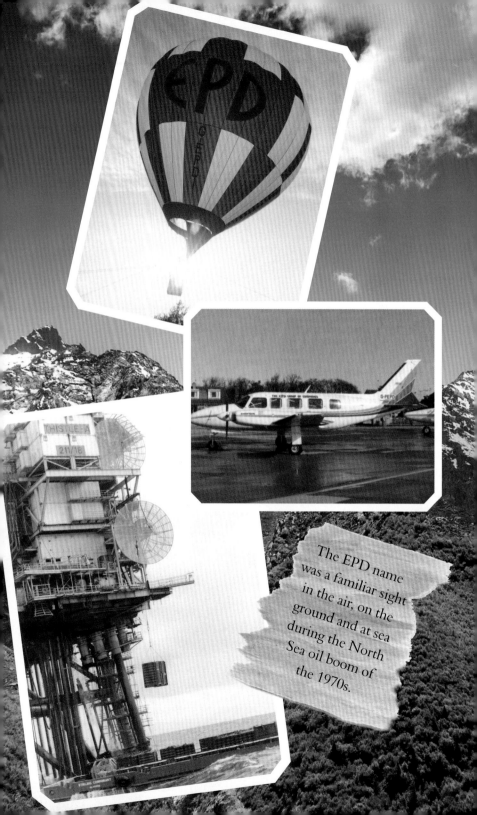

The EPD name
was a familiar sight
in the air, on the
ground and at sea
during the North
Sea oil boom of
the 1970s.

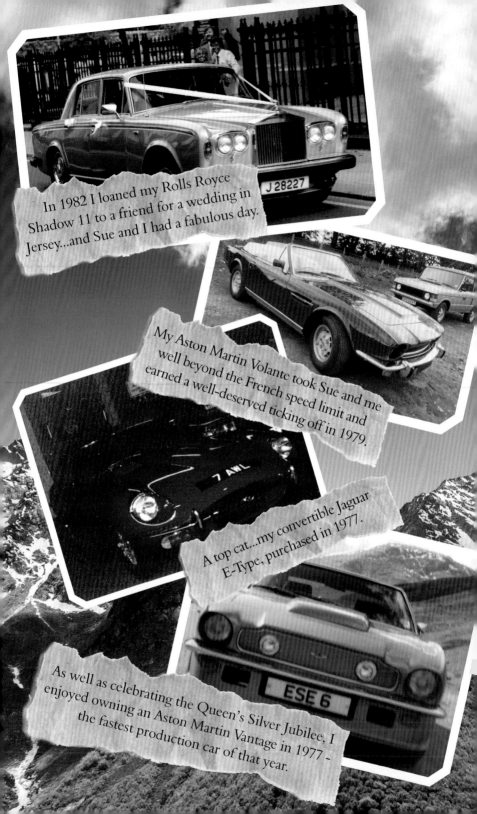

In 1982 I loaned my Rolls Royce Shadow 11 to a friend for a wedding in Jersey...and Sue and I had a fabulous day.

My Aston Martin Volante took Sue and me well beyond the French speed limit and earned a well-deserved ticking off in 1979.

A top cat...my convertible Jaguar E-Type, purchased in 1977.

As well as celebrating the Queen's Silver Jubilee, I enjoyed owning an Aston Martin Vantage in 1977 - the fastest production car of that year.

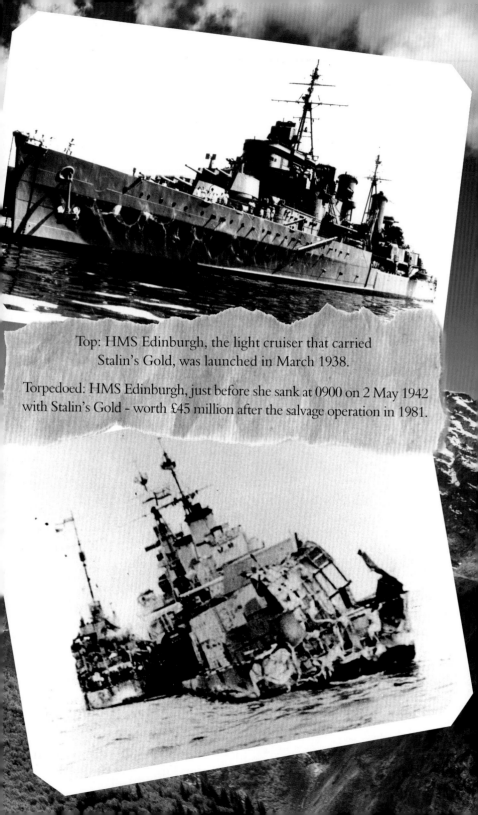

Top: HMS Edinburgh, the light cruiser that carried
Stalin's Gold, was launched in March 1938.

Torpedoed: HMS Edinburgh, just before she sank at 0900 on 2 May 1942
with Stalin's Gold - worth £45 million after the salvage operation in 1981.

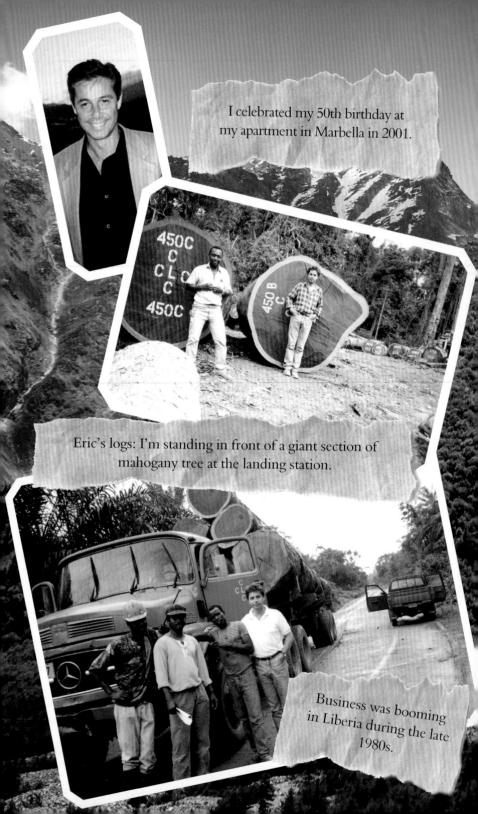

I celebrated my 50th birthday at my apartment in Marbella in 2001.

Eric's logs: I'm standing in front of a giant section of mahogany tree at the landing station.

Business was booming in Liberia during the late 1980s.

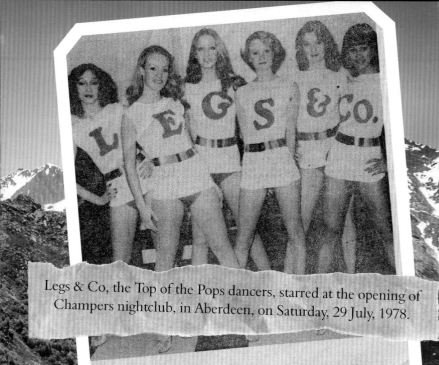

Legs & Co, the Top of the Pops dancers, starred at the opening of Champers nightclub, in Aberdeen, on Saturday, 29 July, 1978.

A cabaret kick-off

☐ CHAMPERS, the Deeside Country Club's nightclub/restaurant, opens its doors at the end of the month.

The club, "designed to provide a service totally neglected in this part of Scotland," intends to provide some top line cabaret in its entertainment.

The opening cabaret act will be Legs and Co., who will appear on July 29. Getting off on the right foot.

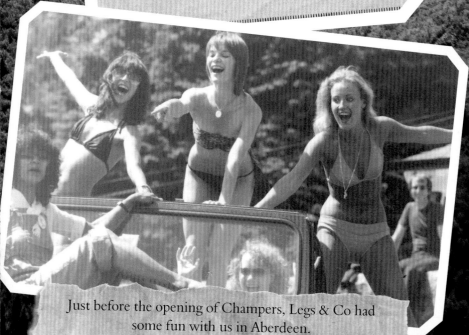

Just before the opening of Champers, Legs & Co had some fun with us in Aberdeen.

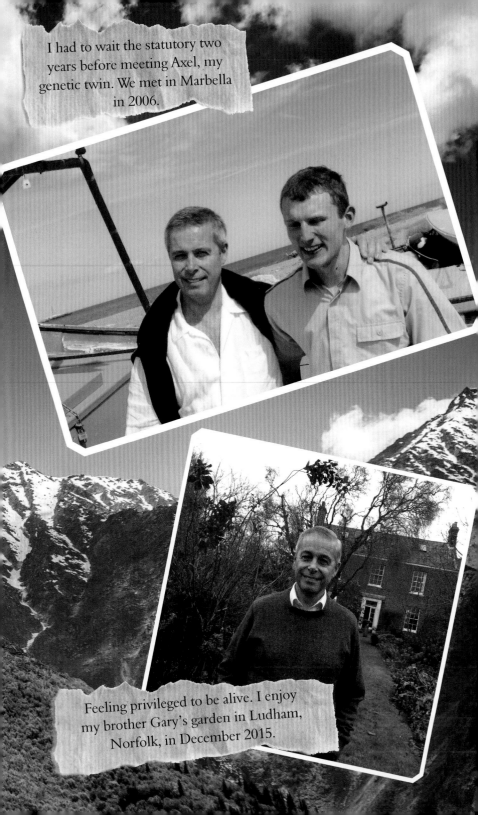

I had to wait the statutory two years before meeting Axel, my genetic twin. We met in Marbella in 2006.

Feeling privileged to be alive. I enjoy my brother Gary's garden in Ludham, Norfolk, in December 2015.

Post donation, Axel will be very tired and spend at least one night in hospital recuperating. As soon as the donation is completed – either today or tomorrow, depending on whether sufficient cells have been harvested – the bone marrow cells will be flown by a medical courier to the UK and delivered to St George's Hospital.

I'm delighted, that apart from a headache, today's medications have been infused much more easily and I've been able to eat and drink properly all day. By the evening I'm feeling much more positive and able to catch up with friends and family on FaceTime and text. I go to sleep wondering how the day has gone for Axel in Dresden, and how he is now feeling. I recall the long chats Axel and I had about those children and their diamonds...

★★★

The day after I met the children at the bush cafe was another manic Monday in the logging business. I had little time to consider the diamonds wrapped in cloth tucked inside my jeans' pocket. At first light the radio buzzed with news from the distant bush, landing station and sawmill more than four hundred miles away.

A seemingly endless list of supplies were 'urgently' required although my idea of urgent was anything that stopped us from operating in the bush – such as fuel and spare parts for machinery – and we usually had those well covered in advance.

Yet again there were problems at Port Greenville. The port captain – a small, thin, frantic local man, demanded backhanders. By mid-morning I was off to Spriggs Payne Airfield to hire one of Quinca's planes. Later in the week I also flew to our logging compound in Grand Gedeh County. The whole time I kept the diamonds wrapped in cloth in my pocket. Occasionally, I reflected on how I would sell them.

Late on the Friday I flew back to Monrovia, arriving just as the sun was setting. How much were my diamonds worth? It was time to find out…

On the Saturday, I returned to the hotel off Benson Street where I had first heard the story about the children and diamonds. The hotel occupied a corner position and the building was old, run down and unloved.

Inside, two young women sat at the bar, seeking attention. Further along the bar, an elderly local man struggled to stand up. At the other end, a group of young Liberian men laughed and joked as they swilled bottle after bottle of local brew. The smell of that odious liquid, mixed with sweat and cigarette smoke, hung over the place like a pungent cloak.

By Liberian standards, the bar wasn't regarded as a seedy place. It was popular with foreigners, day and night. By European standards the establishment was a proper dive.

I positioned myself to obtain a good view of the street outside. There were bright yellow taxis and private cars – ancient imports from Europe – or the occasional new 4 x 4 Mercedes and BMW models. The classier vehicles were driven by a few local wealthy residents or European businessmen.

The colours outside were vibrant, from the street traders in a clash of primary-coloured dresses and wraps, to the endless assortment of eye-catching fruit and vegetables. Back in the bar I watched all the characters chatting and eating, each of them with one end in mind: the next business deal. And, on the outer edge of all this was a mongoose to catch the rats, that chased the cats, which caught the mice; though it seemed that none of them wanted the cockroaches. The entire ensemble scurried around looking for their next meal. I had little choice but to avoid the food on offer and stick to coffee.

I felt in a quandary – wanting to find a dealer for my diamonds, but cautious of alerting anyone to my good fortune. I thought I'd simply wait and see if I recognised anyone.

Everyone knew everyone in the logging business in Liberia; large and small companies were on friendly terms, despite fierce rivalry in the bush. As the owner of Cape Palmas Logging and business partner of Lavoisier Tubman, the ex-President's son, I was certainly known in Monrovia – not only by the people living there, but also by the European buyers. Mostly we dealt with Raab Karcher, a German company who loaned us money and purchased a large proportion of our logs.

Before long, Peter Schroeder from Raab Karcher walked in with a Lebanese man who I didn't recognise.

'Hi,' said Peter. 'Can I get you a drink?'

'A coffee please,' I answered, and then asked the two of them to join me.

Peter was a classic thick-set Bavarian, tall and blond. He lived in Monrovia with his wife and two boys. The two men sat down and Peter introduced Kassim to me.

'I've heard of your company – Peter tells me he buys logs from you.'

We passed the time of day for a while and they ordered a sandwich. With the cockroaches in mind, I politely declined. A few more people came in, some of whom I knew; but Kassim seemed to know everyone. People came over to greet him and it was clear that he was well liked and respected.

'What business are you in?' I asked.

Kassim told me that he had an import and export business with warehouses and trading premises in Waterside, the most prominent commercial district in the capital. Peter excused himself and went over to chat at the bar.

I was left with a stout, well-groomed Lebanese man in his forties who oozed an air of confidence and calmness. I could see it would take a lot to get him flustered. Kassim wore smart shoes, slacks and a designer shirt. He was a cool customer.

'Do you have any contacts who trade in diamonds?' I asked cautiously.

'That's a very interesting question for a man in logging; why do you ask?'

'From time to time I get offered diamonds,' I answered evenly. 'Not many, but I have some now. I can get more – and I'll sell them for cash.'

I certainly had his attention now.

'I'm going back to Waterside,' said Kassim, 'so if you want to come and see me we can discuss this further – say after 4 p.m.?'

I was pleased with the outcome. While I knew nothing about diamonds, I had made my contact, I knew where to find him and he appeared keen to do business.

I left Peter and Kassim at the hotel bar and returned to the house in Sinkor. I checked with the radio operator and all was going well in the bush, landing station and sawmill. There was time for me to have a cup of tea and a chat with Siafa.

Siafa had worked for Lavoisier for a long time; he'd even served his father in office before that. I valued his opinion hugely. We talked for a while and then I brought the conversation around to gold, diamonds and Lebanese traders. He explained that they would buy the diamonds or trade them for goods. The Lebanese community controlled 60% of all trade in Liberia, including most shops, casinos, clubs and bars; they fixed most commodity prices. It was all useful background information for my upcoming meeting.

As the boy opened the gate to let us out, I speculated on the next part of the adventure. The town was busy, especially around the markets in Waterside. The whole area dominated by Lebanese traders. Outside each trader's unit were boxes and sacks stacked high and wide with produce from all over the world.

It all looked chaotic, but in fact everything was highly organised and controlled. The proprietors sat at the front of these shops drinking black coffee in glass mugs, while young boys stacked the shelves and made deliveries. Inside, these shops were crammed with goods across the floor and shelves piled high to the ceiling. It left just enough room to walk to the back office where the real deals were conducted, quietly and in private.

Jerome double parked outside Kassim's shop. As I climbed onto the boardwalk from the kerb, I felt as though I was entering the den of Ali Baba and the Forty Thieves.

I was led through the cavern of goods to the back office where Kassim perched expectantly behind a well-worn old wooden desk. The room was efficiently arranged with endless files on orderly shelves, and papers in trays and neatly stacked samples of goods. There were a couple of seats, plus a substantial sofa and an even more substantial safe. This confirmed to me that I was in the right place.

Someone brought me a coffee, almost chewable, and I sipped it slowly. Kassim said that it had been a pleasure to meet me; he was ready to do business.

'What do you have to sell?' he asked, twirling a pencil in his fingers and eagerly awaiting my response.

I could feel the precious stones pressing against my skin through the pocket of my jeans. There was an obvious bulge where the diamonds lay in wait, ready to attract his eager gaze. Silently, I produced the gems and arranged them neatly on his desk.

Still, I said nothing. The diamonds glinted in the strong light from his desk lamp in the windowless office. There was silence apart from the gentle whirring of the air conditioning fan. Then Kassim stifled a gasp.

'Where were these found?'

'I don't know,' I said. 'But I can have several every two weeks if you're interested. I'm in your hands as to their value. As this won't be a one-off deal it would be good to build a favourable relationship.'

I added that he stocked many items which Cape Palmas Logging bought from other traders and that, if things went well, I would transfer both my business and private purchases to him. That would include bags of rice.

The irony of it all wasn't lost on me. I could see myself buying rice from Kassim, exchanging the grains for the children's diamonds, and then selling the diamonds – to none other than Kassim. I could then visualise Kassim giving me more rice, to trade for diamonds, with the unsuspecting dealer receiving the diamonds from the bush – and giving me cash again! It was so simple. I loved it.

Kassim smiled and I could tell that he was on my side. He told me the rough carat weight of the diamonds and offered me US$600. In 1989 this was perhaps the best price I could get for a metre of prized hardwood loaded onto a ship. The diamond deals had few overheads and vast profits.

I said I wouldn't haggle – though I suspect neither would he – saying that I was in his hands. So that day four rough diamonds, costing me $40 – the American variety – changed hands for fifteen times that amount. I explained that I'd be back from time to time with more diamonds, and he would hear from our people who'd collect the produce we needed on a regular basis. We said goodbye and I left his office with the foul taste of his sticky jet-black coffee in my mouth and 600 greenbacks in my back pocket. In Liberian money that would have been three thousand dollars in 1990.

I settled back into the logging business. As far as I was concerned, though, 'diamonds were forever' and thoughts of future transactions filled my head.

Two weeks later, my diamond day dawned. I awoke early, determined to be on time to meet the children. We left at first light, carrying fifteen bags of rice. The driver successfully negotiated the pot holes on the main road out of Monrovia, and we arrived at the bush trading post at 9.30 a.m. The children were already there, smiling and waving. We parked and they ran to greet us.

I could hardly contain my excitement. They had the same feeling. One of the boys held a dirty grey cloth, and I was absolutely desperate to see the contents. Then he revealed his offerings for the day: four small, shiny diamonds.

At first sight, I thought they only had four, and I was happy to settle for those. However, underneath a corner of the cloth lurked the daddy of them all. This was a huge gem, reflecting light from all angles and capturing my attention in a flash. It glinted in the morning sun, promising a healthy profit from Kassim's Fort Knox safe.

At this time I was consumed by the moment and felt no guilt; that would come only too soon. I enjoyed watching the children drinking their Cokes. They spoke a bizarre form of English, where the sentences ran into each other, almost until the kids ran out of breath. No words were accentuated. But they were beautiful children and I enjoyed our growing relationship. I told them about England, Scotland, my background and my daughters. They loved hearing all about Vicky and Louisa. They became even more excited when I produced pictures of my two girls.

'Why do you want the shiny stones?' queried one of the taller boys.

'I'm taking them to a man In Monrovia,' I answered truthfully, although I knew I was telling only part of the story. 'He's a collector.'

As I gave my economical version of the truth, I thought to myself: 'The rice means nothing to me. The business idea is taking over here.'

We parted soon after that, with promises to meet again in two weeks and waves of goodbye. I left that day thinking more about the children and their families than the diamonds in my pocket. Before long the dusty track met the concrete road heading back to Monrovia and the house in Sinkor.

The logging business soon suppressed my thoughts of the children.

As usual the week was busy, beginning first thing on Monday with a flight in one of Quinca's planes up to the sawmill and landing station; at the end of the week I managed to get to Waterside to see Kassim again. Just as before I was dropped off, but this time I was shown straight through to the office at the back.

'What have you got for me this week, Mr. Eric?'

'Five,' I said, as I reached into my pocket.

'Would you like a coffee?'

'No thanks.'

'A soft drink?'

'Yes, okay. Thank you.'

He took the larger diamond first and examined it intently. The longer he looked, the more interested I became. I asked him what size the diamond was.

'Just under two carats,' he said. '1.8 in fact.'

I waited for Kassim to say his price. He mulled a while and then, as I drank my Coke, he said: 'Three thousand US Dollars for the five diamonds.' The large stone was probably worth considerably more, but I knew nothing about the value of diamonds. I was thrilled to leave Kassim's office with a very healthy return on my investment.

Work in the logging business was as intense and all-consuming as ever. Though Cape Palmas Logging was doing well enough, the company had been in debt to the tune of two million dollars and urgently needed cash to keep on logging. My priority, first and foremost, was to get the Bill of Lading[10] for each shipment presented at a bank, whereupon we'd immediately receive our funds. Logs in the hold meant

10 Bills of Lading are legal documents signed by the carrier and issued to the consignor that evidences the receipt of goods for shipment to a designated person or place.

cash for the company. As a result, I spent much of my time commuting between the Port of Greenville – where I'd pick up the Bills of Lading – and Monrovia, where all the banking was done.

So it wasn't until the Saturday, a fortnight after my previous visit to the bush, that I gave any thought to my excursion the following day. I made sure that I had a good supply of rice and the Range Rover was 'bush ready'.

I was up and away at 6.30 a.m. and, as the gate closed, my mind escaped to the relative relief of my new project. Not even Sue knew about it. As the Range Rover bounced from hole to hole, I was at a loss to understand why successive governments had failed to understand the importance of improving the country's infrastructure.

The road seemed never ending that morning. I heard the occasional "sorry Boss" from Jerome if he miscalculated his speed and the depth of a pot hole. I was feeling physically exhausted and had done so, pretty consistently, since contracting Malaria.

I needed an hour's sleep every afternoon. However, having given my word to the children, I was not about to let them down. I was also keen to check on their haul.

We arrived on time to find the children crouched down in a huddle. As we parked, they came to my side of the Range Rover. When I opened the door we started chatting at once. Jerome made his usual trip to buy Cokes while I entered into gentle negotiations: diamonds for rice again.

This was so far removed from the chaos of running Cape Palmas Logging and my life in Aberdeen or Jersey. Although the children were so young, it felt as if I was catching up with old friends. Spending time with them was becoming a pleasure. I started to see the children as individuals, and they reminded me in so many ways of my daughters.

The children were all excited and obviously proud to let

me know that they'd collected nine diamonds that week, and they carefully opened their white cloth to show me the stones inside. I transferred the diamonds to a black pouch, then Jerome unloaded nine bags of rice.

I explained to them that I would miss the next Sunday and instead be back in four weeks time as I was going home to see my own children. Once more, they asked about Vicky and Louisa and wished me well for the trip.

They waved goodbye and I felt a pang of loneliness as we left them behind. I soon fell asleep, only to be jolted awake by yet another pothole sending a plume of rust-coloured earth in an arc around our vehicle. My mind was now fading from the children in the bush and back to my life in the logging business.

I was due to fly back to the UK with Sue on the Tuesday and had an intense schedule in between to hand over the running of the company in my absence. I remained in Monrovia and managed to see Kassim late on Monday afternoon

After the usual routine with the boardwalk, coffee and Cokes, I pressed Kassim on the political situation. There were rumours about Charles Taylor[11] running riot in Sierra Leone; it would only be a matter of time, I'd heard, before his unwelcome arrival in Liberia.

'It's bad,' he nodded. 'Serious consequences for all of us. I can feel things building up. Our lives are in danger.'

I decided to move the conversation on to the diamonds. I hinted at more success on the diamonds front and produced the black pouch from the side pocket of my jeans.

'Again the smaller ones might not cut well,' Kassim said as his eyes scanned the contents of the pouch.

It sounded like sales talk to me, but that didn't really

---

11 At his subsequent trial by the UN for war atrocities held in The Hague in 2009, it emerged that Charles Taylor had been working with the CIA since the early 1980s, and they were funding his resistance group in 1989.

matter. There were two clear ones, around half a carat each, he told me. He concentrated his gaze on the largest jewel.

'It's the large one that makes the difference, Eric; I will give you three thousand, five hundred US dollars.'

I was always going to accept what he said and showed no emotion as he counted out the money. I never even asked the size of the largest diamond.

Back to the UK, then, for a month away from Cape Palmas logging and diamonds. I enjoyed quality time with Vicky and Louisa and recharged my batteries. The time flew past, and soon enough I was on board a British Airways flight, en route to Monrovia with Sue once more.

There was a palpable difference to the country on our arrival. Passport control was far more stringent than it had ever been before, and there was a noticeable tension as we left the airport with far fewer people out on the streets.

Once home we were greeted by our staff and I sat down with Siafa to go through the good, the bad and the ugly of events from my absence. As usual it was a long list, with many of the problems inevitably requiring a bribe.

On the Saturday Sue and I were up early, when the radio crackled into life as the sun rose in the bush. I listened to updates on the trucks reaching Sinoe and returning for more loads, as well as requests for fuel, spares and food; there was an insatiable demand. We relaxed for the rest of the day, going down to the bar in the hotel in Benson Street and then to the markets in Waterside, where Sue was always happy to browse.

Back at the house, I prepared for my next visit to the bush. I checked that I had a good stock of rice and asked Jerome to make sure that we were fuelled up for the following day. It would be four weeks exactly since my last visit and I was looking forward to seeing the children again.

The routine and the pot holes were exactly the same as before, and we arrived early to wait for the children.

Endless reasons crossed my mind as to why they might not come, but soon enough I spotted six or seven children in the distance, walking in our direction. As soon as they saw us they waved and started running. My eyes filled with tears.

When they arrived, I was sitting on the tailgate. They were genuinely pleased to see us and full of questions about how I was, and if I'd seen my children. There was no talk of Cokes or diamonds; the children were so genuine that I felt quite humble.

As usual I sent Jerome for drinks and asked them all how they were. Pleasantries over, I waited to see the diamonds.

The children were excited and proud, as a white cloth appeared on the tailgate. I was thrilled to see the look on their faces, as they presented their latest collection.

'I found this,' one of the boys grinned.

'Look here at mine,' his friend smiled.

I could barely hide my astonishment as I counted out fourteen diamonds; as we chatted one of the boys produced a stretcher, comprising some fabric lashed to two tree poles. They stacked this home-made device with as many bags of rice as they could, and dragged their prize off behind them. Some of the other children placed the remaining bags on their heads. I was impressed with their ingenuity.

The following weekend, I caught up with Kassim once more. We met for a drink in the hotel bar where Peter had introduced us. After a sociable afternoon, I was three thousand, three hundred dollars better off.

With the children finding more and more diamonds, I was well prepared for my next visit to the bush. We were carrying more bags of rice than before. I imagined that children's bush gossip was all about rice for diamonds; I saw the deal as diamonds for rice. In their own way, they were forging a business in the bush.

'Bossman, too much weight in the back,' Jerome complained as the Range Rover bounced along.

The vehicle was low off the ground, and acceleration took longer than normal. The sun greeted us as we ploughed on along the roughest of roads, kicking up the usual clouds of dust. In the glare of the early morning, my thoughts turned to the children and my growing fondness for them all.

As we approached our destination, I could see my young friends crowded together awaiting our arrival. As soon as we parked, they gathered around us. I counted far more faces than on any previous occasion.

They were all excited. Before long Jerome returned with their drinks and then dropped the tailgate to unload the bags of rice. As I talked and watched the diamonds appear, my eyes were drawn towards a small girl in a deep red dress. She was standing about fifteen metres away and was probably aged four; beside her stood a taller boy of around eight.

They were both looking – in fact staring – at me, and I was so conscious of them that everything else faded out of my sight and hearing. Suddenly all I could see was this boy and the girl who stood out in her scarlet dress, and her direct and unflinching stare. I took a few steps forward and, without hesitation, she walked towards me.

She was so focused that I felt her eyes pulling me towards her. Suddenly there was only the little girl and me, so strong was the determination in her gestures and gaze. Even the young boy seemed to fade away as she approached me, steadfast. Her right arm was motionless and her hand clenched tight. I stood still as she advanced the final few steps. Then, with the boy beside her, she extended her arm, keeping her fist firmly shut.

I was overpowered by her intent gaze and looked intently into her dark eyes. I have no idea how long we were looking at each other; it felt as if time stood still. She continued to say nothing and then eventually she slowly released her grasp and opened up her fingers.

My eyes gradually lowered to her fully-opened hand. In the middle was a large, bright, single diamond. I looked up to her face and she smiled!

Neither of us spoke; no words were needed. Clearly the news of the man who would swap any size diamond for a bag of rice had spread in the bush, and here she was to claim her prize. She was so happy and I understood that pride in achievement; I'd been there myself, many times before.

She gestured towards me and her eyes demanded that I should take the stone. I turned to Jerome and nodded approval for a bag of rice. He brought it over and, for the first time, the girl in the red dress took her eyes off me and looked to her trade – a 28lb of rice. I crouched down and offered the rice with one hand – which the boy beside her accepted – and took the stone from her with the other. I felt numb. It was as though her eyes pierced my very soul.

There was an imprint from the diamond in the skin of her palm; she'd been holding it so tightly. I felt utterly humbled. My driver asked where she was from, and she answered that she'd walked several miles with her brother through the bush. She'd wanted to meet the white man with the rice.

Then all too soon the young boy deftly lifted the bag onto his head and walked back into the bush, hand in hand with the girl in the red dress. A tsunami of emotion overwhelmed me. I had my diamond, but suddenly guilt kicked in. Watching the little girl disappear from sight I felt stripped to the core. And I didn't like what I saw. All those years I'd been chasing the wrong dream, and now a small child in the African bush had humbled my pride. I stood in the dust close to tears.

Jerome passed me a cloth with diamonds wrapped inside but I didn't bother to check how many there were. I simply pushed it into my jeans pocket with my right hand, while I kept the girl's diamond in the other.

As we drove away Jerome remarked: 'Bossman, much better now with no weight.'

I agreed, although with a heavy heart, as I dwelt more on the morality of the transactions. I had no idea how many sacks of rice we'd swapped that day and didn't ask how many sacks we had left.

'The children will be there in two weeks,' Jerome continued. 'They were saying this while you were talking to the girl with the red dress.'

I should have checked myself. I was captivated by Scarlett and her friends, walking miles through the bush for my bags of rice; I was in a world of my own.

It was a long drive back to Monrovia and our house in Sinkor. There was no more conversation. Chris Rea's album 'Road To Hell' played on the radio. My mind was in quiet turmoil.

My Sunday excursions into the bush had become a tranquil escape away from the relentless stresses of the logging industry. The further we drove away from the children, the greater my crescendo of thoughts as I vividly pictured that young child and the indentation of the diamond in her hand. I had no interest in the dollar value of the stone, though I was truly grateful for the lesson in humility.

What had begun as a rumour and turned into diamonds for rice, and then diamonds to dollars, had seemed such a brilliant business adventure. Now I had to completely reappraise my values. A profit; an advantage over the competition in business; being the best. These were the elements that had always been my motivation. Suddenly these little children – and the girl in the red dress – had revealed to me that it is far more important to be of value than to be a success.

Little did I know at the time that I would never see any of

the children again. There would be no more trading diamonds for rice.

I had become a changed man. The few minutes I spent with that small girl one Sunday in the Liberian bush have remained with me, undiminished, ever since.

I will always remember, with affection, the young girl in the red dress, so proudly handing over her prized diamond.

From that moment on, she changed my life. I call her Scarlett.

Yes, Scarlett changed my life for ever.

CHAPTER ELEVEN

Murder in the Night

July 31st 2014. Day nine at St George's Hospital, London.

I wake up feeling so much better than I did yesterday morning and am pleased that, after breakfast, I'm back to my arrival date weight of 66 kilos.

Later in the morning I'm given a blood transfusion in preparation for my transplant tomorrow, and in the afternoon my last infusion of chemo. Everything seems calmer for me, and between meals and routine examinations I'm able to catch up on emails, texts and phone calls.

In the evening I receive an email from Axel letting me know that he is back home from the hospital in Dresden, having been told by the staff that his stem cells were taken by a medical courier on to a London flight.

He ends his email with the words, "I wish you all the best for the next days and weeks. GET WELL SOON MY FRIEND!!!!!" His message brings tears to my eyes. I reply thanking him yet again for his generosity, but my words seem so inadequate in light of his compassion. How can you properly express gratitude for the gift of life?

August 1st 2014. Day ten at St George's Hospital, London, England.

My morning follows the regular routine of four-hourly blood pressure, temperature and pulse readings as well as consuming the contents of a small paper cup containing my eight pills. All the months of medical preparations have been leading up to this day, and I am feeling both excited and anxious at the thought of the transplant.

During the morning I receive two units of blood, and then eat a small lunch while waiting for the transplant, which arrives at 3 p.m. The bag appears larger than ten years ago, and it is a distinct red colour but not as thick as my blood. My new life in a bag from my friend Axel: 291mls with an astonishing 311 million stem cells.

At 3.15 p.m they switch the gravity-fed ball to the 'on' position and the transplant begins. I watch the drips feed down the clear plastic tube through the Hickman Line into my chest where, out of my sight, they enter a large vein just below my right shoulder. The nurses stay with me throughout the thirty five minute process.

From here on it's just a matter of waiting and seeing if the cells engraft in my body and produce red and white blood cells – as well as the vital platelets. This will take between two to three weeks, with the first sign of a successful transplant being the slow rise in neutrophils and platelets. During this time I will take endless pills to stop my body from rejecting the cells. I must sit and wait.

After a couple of hours, a terrible headache develops. I'm given an intravenous drug to make me pass excess liquid, built up from saline solutions. Over the next two hours I pass three litres of fluid, although at the end of that my headache is still severe.

I'm given codeine, which soon works, and then I fall asleep. As I doze off, I return to Liberia once more – and back into the African bush.

★★★

The children in the bush had a profound effect on me. How could I trade a bag of rice for such a valuable diamond? Scarlett was as proud as punch to have the rice; I should have gone to her parents or acted in a more responsible way. I had taken the diamond to boost my finances, when all little Scarlett thought about was eating the rice to survive.

I met up for lunch with Sue and her friends in town and struggled to hide my pensive mood. All around me, people were enjoying the life of privileged ex-pats and my mind kept drifting back to Scarlett.

I left Sue and her friends to their chatting and, by early evening, decided that it was time to head for home. But one of our workers, in town from the bush, asked if we could go for a quick drink at a bar nearby to discuss issues with some of our equipment.

It was a still, warm night, with the stars shining brightly in the tropical sky. We chatted briefly to the English woman who ran the bar and then discussed repairs to a Caterpillar bulldozer. At around 10 p.m. I left the bar to walk the short distance to my house.

The streets were empty and, as I turned into our road, I was immediately stopped by armed police who told me to take an alternative – and much longer – route back home. They gave no reason for their presence, though clearly something serious was going on as I'd never seen roads blocked off by the police before.

When I finally arrived home Sue was already in bed and, not wanting to alarm her, I said nothing. Our house was close to a suburban crossroads. From behind the curtains of my upstairs window I could see police milling about, with many directly outside the house opposite ours. After one last concerned look, I retired to bed.

Early the following morning our peaceful existence in Africa was brought to an end by anguished howls that cut through the dawn chorus. Around two hundred Liberians thronged outside our house, along the street and over the crossroads. Many were shouting, others were crying while some shrieked in dismay. As well as the crowds there were policemen and cars, plus soldiers and army vehicles. We couldn't have opened the gate had we wanted to; there were so many people filling the streets.

Siafa appeared, trying hard to disguise the look of panic all over his face. He told us to stay still, took command of the situation as usual, and forced his way outside to talk to the police and army people. After about twenty minutes he reappeared, still looking alarmed. Although Liberian, Siafa had been educated in America and he could handle a situation from all sides.

'It's serious,' he announced. 'The owner of the house over there had been planning a coup. They killed him.'

'What?' I whispered, realising that danger lurked all around us. 'Killed him?'

Siafa explained that the government, under Samuel Doe, had moved quickly to quash the intended coup. It was clear that Siafa knew a lot more, but he held back in front of Sue. He gestured to go down to the office and I followed, wondering what on earth was coming next.

'Have you heard about being killed in a tribal way?' he muttered as we entered the office.

'I have a good idea,' I admitted.

'The man was murdered in front of his wife and children. It was brutal. There was blood on the ceiling, walls, floor and everywhere.'

'Well, last night something serious was going on,' I recalled. 'We were stopped and told to go home a different way.'

Siafa crumpled into an old, faded leather armchair and stared at me: 'That is when it happened. I talked to people this morning and they said they had heard screams. Now we can see the truth behind all this.'

The murder was a turning point not only for me, but also for Liberia. From that moment nothing would be the same for us – or anyone else in the country. Suddenly, the atmosphere in every area of our lives changed completely. The whole city was on edge and that tension extended wherever I went in the country.

Siafa took complete control of our safety, or as much protection as he was able to provide. He thought Sue was in less danger than me, since he believed that no politician would harm a white woman. He told me that a white man would be targeted for money, and I was certainly no exception.

'You must not go out on your own,' he warned. 'I must know where you are at all times. And you can't go into the bush along with Jerome again.'

'Are you sure?' I pleaded. 'That sounds harsh. I want to go back to…'

'You just do as I say,' Siafa said firmly.

My thoughts sped back to Scarlett and the other children. The thought that I might never see them again was deeply upsetting. The country was on the brink of civil war, he said, and things would only get worse. We had to be on our guard at all times as events seemed to be rapidly escalating out of control; no one knew how bad the situation would become.

From that point onwards there was a heightened military presence throughout Monrovia. Overnight, people became aware that something devastating could occur at any moment. Locals knew only too well about coups and tribal rivalry and eventual revenge. Violence was a frequently trodden path to success in the country – even to the presidency – and everyone felt that the murder of the man in our street was the precursor to large-scale bloodshed.

One name began to be repeated more often than others along with talk of the unfolding disaster: Charles Taylor. He was known to be a Libyan-trained leader of a faction of the army that had turned rebel, operating under the name of the National Patriotic Front of Liberia (NPFL).

Nobody knew exactly what was happening, other than the NPFL had invaded the country from Cote d'Ivoire, and that a multinational West African force, led by Nigeria and assisted by Sierra Leone, had been mobilised to protect Monrovia from the rebels. Doe had come to power through a coup, and now everyone wondered if he would be ousted in the same way.

It was hard to gauge the accuracy of news reports since both the TV and radio stations, as well as the press, were all censored, and much of the news was contradictory. I was in town one day when a car backfired. Instantly everyone crouched down, terrified that the rebels had arrived and hoping that they were not about to be shot.

The atmosphere in Monrovia could be cut with a knife and the main topic of conversation revolved around how everyone would protect themselves. By early 1990 expat families began to leave, slowly at first and then in increasing numbers.

I went into overdrive in my business. Time was definitely not on my side, but I was determined to do my utmost to raise cash. The only way was to load logs onto ships, obtain the Bills of Lading, and then cash those at a bank to pay my creditors. Many of them were small, local traders and I knew that, if I went under, then they would suffer the same fate.

It wasn't long until the start of the rainy season. I could hardly leave hundreds of employees to battle against the elements. And I needed to do my best for the creditors. In any case I had serious money tied up in the business and I would only give up if I was utterly beaten; until then, I'd continue.

My main priority was to get as many cubic metres of logs cut, trucked and loaded on board before the rainy season or the rebels arrived. We'd expanded rapidly and bought new equipment using a $1 million advance from one of our German customers. Repaying that loan each month left us constantly squeezed for cash and now, with a civil war about to erupt on the city streets, all our local suppliers were scrambling around to claim whatever cash was owed to them.

However, with the increasing fear came a decrease in the number of vessels arriving to transport the ever growing mountain of logs accumulating at Port Greenville. Few captains were prepared to take the risk of getting caught up in a coup and potentially having their ship impounded or hijacked by the rebels. The lack of ships docking also led to a drying up of vital supplies and fuel.

There was a burgeoning demand for US dollars by certain individuals and government departments. While bribery had always been prolific, it now went stratospheric. If it wasn't the port captain it would be an FDA official demanding payment to allow our logs to be loaded. Everyone from the top of Doe's government to its lowest ranks was in a desperate scramble to extort US dollars in any and every possible way. I felt trapped in the eye of a financial storm.

Aside from the pressures of business there was also the uncertainty over civil unrest in an African country, noted for atrocities. I had never previously been afraid of anyone, be it a person or situation. Now, I became literally sick with fear. I knew that I was in the wrong place at the wrong time. I was violently sick every morning.

One frantic day in Monrovia, while I was struggling with the demands of creditors and import/export issues, I took a break and consoled myself with a coffee in a local café.

I paid and walked out, only to be confronted by two men in military uniforms, looking as if they owned everything and everyone in the neighbourhood. An arrest and interrogation session appeared to be imminent.

'This looks serious,' I muttered to Jerome. 'Take the Range Rover back to the office and tell Siafa I've been arrested.'

'Get in,' the more officious of the two ordered as a yellow taxi ground to a halt outside the café. The lumbering old Toyota lurched towards the Executive Mansion.

'Get out,' the same official-looking military man snarled when we arrived.

I was escorted to the third floor where another two men, decorated to the hilt, were waiting for me.

One of the strutting pair wore a sweat-stained jacket, packed with buttons and braids. Judging by the man's harsh face and tone, and rivulets of sweat, he looked in no mood for negotiation. The room had no air conditioning; the place stank, and the soaking armpits confronting me did little to clear the air.

'How do you plead?' he barked.

'I have no idea what you are talking about, so I plead not guilty.'

At this stage I was becoming more and more anxious. I thought it was a case of everyone in power trying to extract money wherever they could as the rebels caused havoc in the bush. He repeated the question and I answered in the same way.

'How about a few hours in our jail downstairs? That might change your mind. I am charging you with economic sabotage. How do you plead?'

''Not guilty.'

The two men looked at each other. 'Okay, strip down to your pants and stand there while a charge sheet is prepared,' said the sweating man with the buttons and braids.

His skinny colleague sat down at the desk and took several pieces of paper with accompanying carbon sheets and threaded them into an ancient Olivetti typewriter. He banged the keys slowly to make sure that the letters went through to each sheet. The keys stuck to the ribbon and became entangled. He released them and tried again as I assumed he was typing out my death sentence.

The painfully slow typing, with the tangled letters, seemed to ratchet up the tension. The official who was charging me appeared to be edging ever closer to breaking point. I just stood in my underpants, watching the cockroaches scurrying around, and trying to remain calm.

Finally, the senior officer pulled out his gun from its

holster, pointed it my head and said: 'Are you still saying you're innocent of economic sabotage?'

Before I could answer, the door burst open and in stormed another military man, more buttoned and braided than my interrogator. The garbled language told me that he was second-in-command to Doe. The unexpected visitor was tall, sweating profusely, and looked in total panic mode.

He gave me a cursory glance and then blurted out: 'He's shot him!'

My inquisitor looked stricken and lowered his gun while his nervous colleague behind the typewriter appeared terrified. I had no idea to what or to whom they were referring, but I was gripped with fear. Then the story came tumbling out and I realised that I had, coincidentally, been witness to its inception.

A couple of days earlier, Sue and I had been in a bar close to our house on the Sinkor road where all the expats gathered. We'd been chatting with friends when an American who worked at the embassy came over and asked if we wanted to go with him to another bar in the centre of the city. He was well on the way to being pretty drunk so we declined and thought no more of it.

A while later he suddenly burst in, shouting that he'd been shot. We thought he was joking until he pulled down his sock and showed us the hole in his foot with a bullet lodged deep inside. He explained that the taxi taking him into town had passed a new checkpoint manned by an unpaid military youth high on cane juice – the local firewater. The drunken young officer had tried to stop the car by firing at its front tyre. The bullet missed the tyre, and instead passed through the passenger door into the American's foot. The woman behind the bar immediately took him to hospital and we heard no more about it after that.

Back in the interrogation room, the rest of the incident was revealed. Shortly after being admitted to hospital, the

American Ambassador to Liberia asked the patient whether he wanted to be med-evacuated back to the States. The alternative was having the bullet removed in Monrovia. The young American trusted the Liberian surgeons. He was taken down to the theatre, given too much anaesthetic, and died on the operating table.

Clearly the Ambassador had made a complaint. On hearing about the American's death Samuel Doe had gone down to the jail in the Executive Mansion and asked the gunman to identify himself. A horror-struck boy of no more than twenty stepped forward.

'Did you shoot the American?' demanded the President.

'Yes,' replied the startled youth.

Without a further word Doe had pulled out his gun, lifted it to the boy's temple, pulled the trigger and shot him dead.

This was all witnessed by Doe's second-in-command, who was now in the room with my interrogators. Shocked by the appalling account, I was ready to admit to almost anything and pay up.

'What's going on here?' asked the recently arrived, highly decorated and highly sweaty newcomer.

The confused looking group spoke for a while in whispers. Perhaps with one dead American, and one dead Liberian, events were making them pause for thought.

Suddenly the phone on the desk rang. Doe's number two took the call and then I was hastily told to get dressed. The charge sheets of paper and carbon copies were ripped out of the typewriter and thrown in the bin. I had no idea if I was heading to jail or being released without charge onto the streets; I said nothing.

I was escorted downstairs where, to my relief, Siafa was waiting with Willy Givens, the Liberian Ambassador to Britain. Willy was an old friend who just happened to be in Monrovia at the time of my arrest. Siafa had had the presence of mind to call him to plead my case. With my wallet emptied of several thousand Liberian dollars and stress levels off the scale, I was released without charge.

We all went back to the bar where a few hours previously I'd been arrested outside, and had a few drinks while I slowly unwound. Siafa was full of apologies for my treatment, embarrassed by the behaviour of some of his countrymen. After a while we left and the day returned to its usual pattern. Later on, when I returned home, I played down the incident and explained to Sue that it had all been a misunderstanding. By that point, we had already had many conversations about Sue leaving Liberia, but she was adamant that she wouldn't go without me. I'd given up on trying to persuade her otherwise, and didn't think there was any point in frightening her with the details of my horrific ordeal.

As I undressed for bed, I noticed some bulges in my trouser pockets. I hadn't been searched properly. I was amazed to find the large diamond from Scarlett, and the diamonds from the other children, still in my clothing. That would have taken some explaining!

The arrest compounded my fear. In the bush, my workers were absolutely terrified. The fighting was drawing ever closer. The rebels could arrive and rape, maim or kill my workers and their families at any moment.

With the mounting tension came growing lawlessness, though more so in town than the bush. Old scores were being settled as ethnic tensions rose. I still felt safer in the bush than anywhere else.

At the house I was awoken daily by noisy creditors outside the gate. Some of them screamed my name; the pressure was mounting. Time was running out to transport logs and sawn timber to the port, and even fewer vessels were docking in Greenville. My only chance of financial survival lay in obtaining a substantial payment from a Bill of Lading.

In the days that followed we worked tirelessly to empty all the logging stations, cut as much sawn timber as we could with the fuel we had left, and transported it all to the port. We pulled all the equipment – the two Caterpillar skidders, the road grader, Bedford and fuel trucks – back to the sawmill, and shut down the bush operation.

I circled the bush and port by air for an overview of the situation, and then spent several days driving continuously between the sawmill and Port Greenville. At the same time, our trucks drove back and forth, night and day.

Finally, we transported all our stock to the port and I was determined to get the logs and sawn timber on board the next vessel – due to arrive in two days.

The port was brimming with timber from all the various logging companies. I was determined to make one last shipment so that I could settle with creditors – if not all of them, then at least most.

All the logging companies knew of this vessel's impending arrival, and of course everyone wanted their logs loaded on board first. The ship would have a sizable capacity – but it couldn't take the mountain of logs that all the different companies had built up in and around the port: some timber would have to be left behind and I was determined they wouldn't belong to Cape Palmas Logging.

I had prepared all the paperwork, cleared it with the port captain and asked him for the order of loading. He kept his answer vague, saying everyone wanted their logs loaded first. Nevertheless he assured me that my logs would make the sailing and, having paid the man a small fortune over the years, I was confident that he would honour his word.

The following morning, down at the port, I saw the high wheelhouse of the most derelict, rust-ridden tub I'd ever seen arrive at the dock. However, it was massive – around five hundred feet long – taking up the entire length of the dock, and clearly had a huge capacity for carrying cargo. Despite my scepticism that it could sail up the coast, let alone to Europe, all I had to do was get my logs on board. Then I would be presented with Bills of Lading, which I could instantly turn into cash at a bank. The end of a huge source of stress was finally in sight.

I had already arranged the sale of the timber for US$500,000 with our largest buyer in Germany, who had loaned us money. Our agreement was that they would keep 50% of the Bill of Lading value, which meant there was $250,000 to come to Cape Palmas Logging. The vast majority would go straight to creditors, while I was going to keep back $10,000 for myself, even though at that point I was owed far more by the company.

As it drew up, the vessel slammed into the quay, adding yet another dent in its buckled side. Ropes were cast and the proverbial motley crew appeared on deck. I walked up the gang plank and was shown to the captain's cabin. He turned out to be Dutch and we drank a Beck's together while the port captain and customs officer cleared the boat for arrival into port, Liberian style.

I had only one thing in mind – my logs on board at any cost. The moment the vessel was moored, trucks lined up along the dock, ready to offload. Further along, caterpillar machines tipped logs into the water to be floated by 'swimmers'. The ship's three cranes hovered expectantly, ready to grab enormous amounts of cargo from the waterside. The vessel's cargo holds were vast and empty. I estimated that it would take two to three days, working round the clock, to complete loading. The harbour was, all of a sudden, a hive of activity.

When I stepped off the vessel the port captain immediately came over to me and said that our logs were on hold; he didn't know why but I had to see the FDA personally in Monrovia to receive clearance.

I was fuming, but had no option other than to radio for one of Quinca's planes to collect me. A few hours later

I was back in Monrovia where Jerome took me directly to the FDA office. The official there just grinned when I walked in. He was immaculately dressed, officious, and I could tell that he was holding all the cards. The FDA's top man was livid when I asked why he'd put Cape Palmas' logs on hold.

'You owe the FDA money in back taxes,' he said.

'That is nonsense,' I retorted.

'You must pay $16,000,' he continued. I knew he meant Liberian dollars, but it was still a substantial sum.

Again, this was untrue although I said we would check it out and pay anything we owed, but asked that the logs be loaded in the meantime.

He just smiled, looked at me, and waited for my offer. I was close to exploding, but instead managed to stay calm and explained my plight. I offered to make him a contribution of $2,000, showing my appreciation of his position.

He kept me in suspense for a minute or two before picking up the phone to the port captain in Greenville. 'Eric's cleared to go,' he said.

I kept my cool, thanked him, and grudgingly handed over the bribe. I'd come well prepared with $1000 in each of four pockets. He had no idea that I was prepared to give him twice as much. I made it back to Port Greenville by Quinca's plane just as the sun was setting. Dark clouds loomed above me: the rainy season had arrived.

Finally cleared for loading, I approached the port captain. I needed clearance to bring my trucks in line.

'Well, it's like this Eric, I've been told to get these companies' logs loaded first,' he said.

'Mine have far fewer cubic metres and will take only a small space.' I pleaded.

'My hands are tied, Eric. I can do nothing more. You just have to wait and see what space is left.'

At that point I calmly lost it. Without another word I left his office, told my drivers to form their trucks in a new line alongside the port-cleared trucks, and walked onto the quayside. By then it was dark, torrential rain had begun, and floodlights had been switched on.

A mighty Caterpillar grab was loading logs from trucks onto the quay before they were swallowed up by the vessel's cavernous holds. The mighty machine picked up a load of five 50ft logs and advanced at almost 20mph towards the vessel. I stepped directly in front of the Caterpillar and put my hands up. The driver, about twenty feet above me in his cabin, could do nothing but abruptly stop the fifty-ton behemoth. High above me the logs rocked noisily in their cradle and the Caterpillar's tyres, much taller than me, bulged with the braking while the rain soaked me to the skin. Everything stopped.

I watched the port captain surveying the scene from his vehicle. He seemed at a loss about what to do. He scanned the long line of logging trucks as though he required their permission for his next move.

Most of these logging companies had massive funds behind them, some had dubious money, and they were not to be messed with. However, at that moment I was standing up for my principle: he had given me his word and I would not be moved or beaten.

Before long another logging boss beckoned the port captain over. I felt so alone, wet, exhausted, scared and in fear of my life, but completely driven. I stood my ground, with my hands in the air for about five minutes, by which time I was close to tears. Finally the port captain walked over.

'Okay, you win Eric, bring all your trucks in, and we will load you now!'

The hulking Caterpillar backed off and dropped its load on the quay. No one could see, but silent tears ran down my face as I waved my trucks to come in and overtake the long line of my competitors.

It took hours, but we emptied our yard that night. I watched the whole process from my 4 x 4 truck parked at a distance, with the rain teeming down the entire time. The port captain eventually admitted that two of the other logging bosses had bribed their way to loading first, but I was the only other logging owner who stood up to them. Whether I was foolish or brave is questionable, but there would be no logs in my yard when the vessel left Port Greenville. The other logging bosses may have been mean and ruthless, but at least I had earned their respect.

As the sun rose the following morning I was able to conclude my business and collect the Bills of Lading, worth $500,000 – US dollars this time – ready for my departure with Quinca's plane later that afternoon. I thanked all my truck drivers and engineers who maintained the engines, and wished them a safe journey back into the interior. I knew it would be a final farewell. No one, not even Sue, had any inkling that this would be my last ever visit to either the bush, sawmill or port. I was in a fearful retreat.

As Donald Trump said: 'Part of being a winner is knowing when enough is enough. Sometimes you have to give up a fight and walk away, and move on to something more productive.'

That time had definitely come. I could fight all the difficulties of the logging industry, but not those of a coup. Problems were escalating and I felt almost constantly in fear for my life. After my numerous arrests I knew that, as a logging company owner, I was a target for bribery, and perhaps even butchery. From world news bulletins we knew that the rebels were advancing towards Monrovia from the north, and I was not going to be there, sitting out the rainy season. By then we were among the very few expats remaining in the country and, along with most of the others still there, I was planning our escape.

I left the house in Greenville full of sadness, remembering the good times with Sue, the mongoose and the monkey, and the long dusty drive up to the virgin bush and the heart of our business. Tamba, our driver based in the bush, took me down to the port for a final time. It was eerily quiet after the swarming of trucks and driving rain, and my stance on the dock the previous evening.

The port captain stopped his car for a chat. We had a respectful conversation, reflecting on the traumatic events during loading. I had a few hours to kill before Quinca's pilot was due at the airstrip and hung around and watched as the insect-killing chemical bombs were dropped into the holds. Eventually the gigantic log-carrying vessel departed, limping and listing, for its arduous voyage to Europe.

I asked the driver to take me around our storage yard outside the port gates. All that was left were the imprints from where our pyramid of logs had sunk into the scorched red earth and the tracks from our vehicles. Spindly bark strands littered the yard; the only remains of our logs as they lumbered onwards to Europe.

I went into the village nearby, bought a beer in the hut of a shop, and sat in a rickety chair outside. I watched the world go by, wondering if I'd ever see the bush, the port or my employees again. It was surprisingly peaceful. How long would that peace last?

Children played in the dust next to the street and I bought them all a Coke, much to their surprise. Of course they took my mind back to Scarlett and the other children in the bush some five hundred miles away. I felt sad that I wouldn't be able to say goodbye to them and was fearful for their safety too. I hoped that, by some miracle, they would be able to evade the rebel troops.

It was soon time to go. Fearing the unknown, and feeling depressed at my unsuccessful business endeavours, I was driven for the final time to the grass airstrip a few miles above Port Greenville. It had always been one of my favourite places in Liberia, where I'd stroll along the airstrip on the dusty grass elevation while I waited for one of Quinca's planes; there were no phones, fax machines or incessant voices demanding to be heard.

Tamba offered to stay with me, but I told him to return to the bush camp.

'Take care,' I said, and we both knew that was the end of the road for us.

'Bye Boss,' he whispered softly as he drove away. My heart was in my mouth at that moment.

The airstrip was deserted and the fierce heat of the day subsided as the setting sun turned red. I stood waiting for Quinca's aircraft, feeling sad and alone. I took solace in thinking of Vicky and Louisa and what they might be doing. I took comfort that I had the Bills of Lading in my briefcase – my creditors would be paid.

As I watched the setting sun, two eagles came into view about a hundred feet above me. They were playing and so obviously carefree, oblivious to all the problems in the country below them. They seemed to represent all that was good in the world – nature untouched by man. I thought about my own impact on the virgin bush. At least the rains would soon wash away the roads and bridges we'd built, and I hoped that the FDA had in fact used the vast fees we'd paid them to replant the forests. Perhaps, I thought, the bush would devoir newly-opened spaces and destroy any trace of our activities.

Gradually the distant drone of a plane filled the sky and the eagles flew away. I waited at the end of the runway, trying to enjoy my last moments in Greenville and imprint a picture of the place on my memory. I saw the plane approaching in the distance and watched as it grew from a speck to a four-seater aircraft.

Quinca's ageing Cessna landed with the sun behind, and

soon pulled up beside me. I took one final look around before I opened the door and jumped in.

As we increased our speed down the runway I decided not to look back. I just kept watching the vast, red sun as it rested for the night, somewhere over the Atlantic Ocean.

All at once, I felt a sense of freedom. I felt as free as those eagles, soaring high in the night sky.

I was totally unprepared for the turbulence to come.

CHAPTER TWELVE

The Diamond that Saved My Life

August 2nd 2014. Day eleven at St George's Hospital London.

I wake after a reasonable night's sleep and am pleased to be able to eat breakfast. I still take pills every evening to help me sleep; that way the days pass quicker with less time to fill. Today is a day off medication, though the four hourly check-ups continue and I have my regular blood test.

One day into the transplant, and I ask myself how long it will take to engraft, and I spend much of the day thinking about all that has happened since my first transplant. It is much easier this time, having contact with Axel and knowing what he's going through.

August 3rd 2014. Day twelve at St George's Hospital.

Today I begin a course of Lenograstim, which I will receive until engraftment has taken place. I'm feeling much better. Throughout the day Vicky and Louisa are on my mind. Their lives carry on while mine is, in some ways, on hold. It makes me so happy that they are well and settled; I look at my photos of them and smile. I spend some of the day catching up with phone calls and emails, and let Axel know how the transplant has gone. In the evening I receive the following email in reply to mine:

"Dear Eric,

I had looked forward so much for your email. Thank you!!!!!

I was a little bit afraid if everything works well. Nice to hear that you had a good night after transplant. I think of you every day and hope all the time that everything goes well. After donation the nurse in Dresden show me the bag with stem cells and I saw your name and the hospital St George's written on it. I took the bag on my heart and wish all the best for you.

Great to hear from you.

Best wishes my friend,

Axel"

What can I say about this mature soul in a young man's body? Words really fail me, but he is like my guardian angel: always there for me when I need him, just as he promised ten years ago.

Happy to hear from Axel, my mind drifts back to my past adventures – and that emotional flight from Port Greenville back to Monrovia.

★★★

Quinca's pilot asked if I wanted to fly the plane when we took off from Greenville, but I declined, unusually for me. I was hardly in the right frame of mind; instead, I recounted the bizarre series of events while I watched the setting sun, with a kaleidoscope of dazzling colours in the evening sky. I kept my thoughts to myself as day turned to night and the aircraft flew on beneath thousands of twinkling stars.

Little did I know that a large, twinkling uncut diamond and a bag of rice would shape my future and help to propel me out of Liberia.

It had been an exhausting few days and, although I finally

felt relaxed and so pleased that our logs had been loaded against all odds, I knew that the following few weeks were likely to be more than difficult. Flying towards Monrovia, I was as free as those eagles. No one could call me, walk in, arrest me, or even just see me. Only Sue, my staff in the bush and in town knew of my whereabouts.

Gradually the lights of Monrovia appeared in the distance. As they grew brighter my feelings of turmoil and apprehension returned. We landed in a screech of tyres and were soon parked at the hangar. Jerome collected me and drove back to the house.

He warned: 'Boss man, lots of people looking for you today, all waiting at the gate to see you.'

It wasn't what I needed to hear, though it didn't surprise me. I tried to clear my head, had a bite to eat with Sue, and plunged into the comfort of bed.

I slept in until 7 a.m., a little later than usual, but I was mentally shattered. I rushed to the bathroom and was immediately sick as usual. It was a horrible way to start the day; however the fear and dread would not subside. At least my hard-won Bills of Lading would soon resolve many of my most immediate, pressing problems.

All was well when I checked in the radio room; the trucks had returned to camp without incident and everyone there was safe. For that I was thankful. Again the tiny birds on the tree outside the office brought a smile to my face. Siafa was already there and told me that people had been queuing outside since 6 a.m.

'All in good time,' I said. 'I'm off to the bank.'

'Well done!' he answered with a broad smile.

As the gate opened for Jerome, the crowd surged around us, fists in the air and shouting. We sped off quickly towards town and the bank.

Central Monrovia was a whirl of activity. The bank seemed even more so, with everyone shouting, pushing, and demanding attention. Thankfully the manager saw me and beckoned me into his office. I felt as though I'd been rescued from the fray. The noise dimmed as he closed the door. I was offered tea and we talked about the growing unrest and the flight of most expat families. I then produced my Bills of Lading and asked him to release the agreed $250,000 to the buyer, and to give me the balance in cash. He smiled and gave the documents to his clerk.

From the bank I planned to go to Waterside for a favourable rate of exchange – seven or eight Liberian dollars to one USD. I would change about $150,000 to around a million Liberian dollars. That would be more than enough to cover everything. The Liberian dollar was worth less and less as days drew on.

The clerk said that the transaction, release of funds, and count of US dollars would take about an hour.

'I'll call back then,' I said, quickly finished my tea and left the bank.

I decided to spend the time in a café in Benson Street, where a thousand thoughts raced through my mind. Would I be arrested again, outside the café? Would I have enough money to pay everyone? Was the fighting intensifying?

Break over, I returned to the bank with a slight spring in my step and was immediately shown into the manager's office.

'We have a problem,' he said, sternly. 'The buyer has taken all $500,000 against his account, and though he confirms the arrangement you made, he has reneged on it. There is nothing I can do.'

I was speechless. The news hit me like one of the North Sea's rearing gale force twelve storms. It took several minutes for me to even speak while I was shuffled out of the manager's office. I asked to use one of the bank's phones and dialled the number of the buyer in Germany. I was surprised when I got through.

'I cannot believe what I've just heard,' I said. 'Is it true? You gave me your word.'

'My hands are tied, Eric, there's nothing I can do. I am just an employee and it's not my decision.'

It was as if he was repeating the port captain's message of doom. Enough was enough, surely. Donald Trump's words resonated in my head as I hovered over the abyss.

'Please release just $50,000.'

'I cannot.'

'$40,000.'

'Sorry. It's more than my job's worth.'

We got down to $10,000 and I stopped. I was begging now and he sat at his desk in Dusseldorf just saying 'no' and waiting for the humiliating conversation – from my point of view at least – to end. The company had made us the loan and, with the impending civil war, obviously wanted to claw back as much of it as they could, irrespective of any agreement.

Not a dollar passed to me that day. I felt exhausted, deflated, sick, and desperate with mounting panic at the thought of going back without the money.

I walked downstairs from the first floor of the bank to the bustling street below. It was a struggle to actually walk. My legs refused to move and I slumped against the wall. How could I go back to the office? What would I say? No one would believe the story, certainly not a creditor. I needed time to think, decide what to do and make a plan. That was easier said than done with no money and just words, but I would have to come up with something. I told Jerome to park up and then meet me in an hour's time at the café in Benson Street. I needed time to re-assess and adapt before moving forward.

Once at the cafe, I ordered a large vodka and tonic. It seemed an age since I'd waited for the plane, watched the eagles and enjoyed the sunset. What a difference a day can make.

I looked at my photos of Vicky, Louisa and Sue and smiled as though I hadn't a care in the world. They're what really matters, I thought; you don't die from this! I went through my wallet as though I might find a miracle inside: there were a few US and Liberian dollars, a couple of credit cards, and some receipts and scraps of paper with phone numbers. It provided a brief distraction and took my thoughts back to my daughters in Aberdeen.

From there my mind drifted to the children in the bush and I surprised myself as I'd forgotten about the diamonds in my jeans pockets. I could see the cloth sticking out of one pocket, and felt the other one to check for Scarlett's diamond. Thankfully, it was still there. But it was time to deal with more urgent matters.

I paid the bill, left the cafe, jumped in the Range Rover and asked Jerome to take me back to the house. My heart was in my mouth as we neared home. When we reached the gates the crowd's impatience had turned to open hostility. It took several minutes just to get through the gate, with the horde hammering on the vehicle and hollering for money.

Finally safe inside the gates, I explained the situation to Siafa. He offered to talk to them. That was a painful job for me – and me only. I understood that the situation for almost all of them was awful; I had no money to hand over, but at least I could give them my time.

Siafa opened the gate and announced that I would see everyone individually. It took the rest of the day and the range of reactions was vast. Some of the creditors were calm and understanding, while others simply didn't believe the events at the bank. There was shouting, banging on the table, near violence and threats of attack. Some refused to leave until paid – clearly a futile protest.

I really felt the pain of the smaller creditors, who were clearly in most need – and yet generally they showed the most understanding and belief in my plight. At the end of it all, I was done in. I could scarcely believe how matters had descended so quickly into such chaos: all the consequences of an impending coup.

What would those consequences be?

A few days later Siafa burst into the radio room with the news that a military vehicle, filled with soldiers, was approaching the house. Minutes later the house was surrounded with armed soldiers, the gates were forced open, and the commander burst into Siafa's office. We could hear him shouting at the top of his voice. He pushed open the door to the radio room, where Siafa and I were waiting, frozen to the spot.

'I have a warrant for the arrest of Eric Evans and a court order to shut down Cape Palmas Logging,' he snarled. 'Everyone must leave the premises now. The building will be locked and guarded and no one can return.'

My heart sank as it beat faster. As I stood up two soldiers came to stand either side of me. Lavoisier Tubman arrived on the scene and used every tactic and important name he knew to halt my arrest. At that point, Sue walked into the room and I told her to go to a friend's house with some overnight clothes; this was all just a misunderstanding and I would sort it out in town.

Everyone was removed from the house that day, and once again I was escorted to the Executive Mansion. I was taken to a bleak room and questioned about Cape Palmas Logging and, in particular, the Bill of Lading for $500,000, which the company had not been paid out on. This time there was no request for cash, and I realised that they believed I was funding someone – possibly supporting rebels – with the sale of logs. I could understand, from their questioning, how it could look that way.

A splinter group from Charles Taylor's NPFL, led

by Prince Johnson,[12] another military man turned rebel, was now just days away from Monrovia. His propaganda machine made it widely known that the first targets in the city would be Samuel Doe, his armed forces, and all expatriates. The men questioning me wanted answers – fast.

Lavoisier and Siafa produced the paperwork, proving the non-payment of the Bills of Lading, including the reasons why the money had not come through. The government's only concern was to keep funds out of Johnson's reach. The marauding prince was funded through conflict diamonds. Now his opponents believed that he was about to receive vast sums through conflict logs.

That was the darkest day of my life, before or since. For seven long hours I stared into the face of untold horrors.

The sweaty commander, braided to the hilt, yelled: 'Admit it. Where is the money? Who are you supporting? The rebels?'

'The bank didn't give me any money,' I insisted. 'Look, you can…'

'Liar!', his gun toting companion spat. 'We are running out of patience. The truth, please.'

'I am telling the truth,' I repeated over and over again. 'The paperwork is correct.'

Reluctantly, snarling and sweating from every pore, the pair of panicky looking soldiers had a longer read of the paperwork. I was in the clear – just.

When I was finally released I felt that I had been tipped from turmoil into a black hole. While I'd already made my mind up to leave the country, the time for my departure had unequivocally arrived.

I was handed over to Siafa and Lavoisier who both echoed my thoughts. Lavoisier had served in the government prior to

---

12 The name Prince is a common given name in Africa, as is the case here, and does not refer to a title.

Doe's coup several years beforehand. He escaped the ensuing massacre and knew what lay in store this time.

I asked them both to keep my plans secret, even from Sue. Any hint of my impending departure would surely lead to another arrest with a dubious outcome. I was a marked man, despite my innocence being reluctantly accepted.

We collected Sue from her friend's house. I could barely speak but managed to explain the day away as yet another misunderstanding between the government and Cape Palmas Logging.

Back home, still saying little, I sank into bed. Sue kept asking me what was going on, but I continued with my stories about misunderstandings. My mind lurched from one disaster to another. After a fitful sleep I awoke at 6 a.m., hurried through to the bathroom, and was violently sick as usual.

Three hours later Lavoisier arrived with Gihad Ghiada, who was a co-shareholder in Lavoisier's 49% of the company.

'I do not want you to leave,' Gihad told me firmly.

I was taken aback. Lavoisier had told me he could get all his co-shareholders to support the decision for me to leave. Now Gihad was bluntly threatening to tell the authorities if I tried to escape. He wanted $8,000 – the valuable America versions – to enable him and his family to leave, and not a dollar less. I was speechless, and my shock and fury were plain to see.

'Why should you get out and not me?' he reasoned. That was a fair point, although I wasn't looking to him to find money for my escape, or threatening to tell the authorities about his plans.

Lavoisier, always a gentle man, was close to losing his temper at this point, but I stopped him. Gihad's trump card was that he could get airline tickets for Sue and me from a relative who worked in a travel agency; they would also be able to keep my name off the passenger list. I had one chance to get out. The next and last flight was scheduled for the coming Friday at 9 p.m. Airlines were closing their Monrovia routes from that day onwards because of the troubles.

Until then, I hadn't given any thought as to how I would actually leave Liberia. But it suddenly dawned on me that I wouldn't be able to just book a flight and get on a plane – my name on any departure list would ensure my arrest. Clearly Ghiada understood his position of strength and there was no point in trying to reason with the man. I agreed to his terms, not knowing how I'd pay him or find the money to buy tickets.

Later that day, more details of chaos crackled out of the receiver in the radio room. News had spread like wildfire. Prince Johnson and his rebels were on their way, murdering and maiming en-route.

As a result Monrovia itself was in turmoil, full of desperate, scared and violent people, many of whom would do absolutely anything – from looting, to stealing, extorting, or even murder – to leave Liberia.

My mind returned to Vicky and Louisa in Aberdeen, and I was thankful for their safety. My thoughts also returned to Scarlett and the other children in the bush; I prayed that they had avoided disaster.

Then, a brainwave: Scarlett's diamond.

In that instant a weight was lifted from me. The diamonds might yet save my life. I had to get to Kassim, and quickly.

I was keeping Siafa informed of my every move and told him that I had to go into town. He looked at me intently and must have seen that I had a serious purpose in mind.

'Go directly where you need to go and then come back immediately,' he urged.

'Okay,' I smiled.

With an impending coup on the way, no fuel was coming into the country. Liberia was the last place a cargo ship would dock. Fearful anticipation gripped the population.

The few people outside looked at the rare sight of our black Range Rover with unease, assessing whether or not they might have to suddenly run for their lives. It was all unnerving. Even in the city centre the normal throngs had vanished and the market was now like a ghost town, apart from a few brave market traders. Waterside was deserted as we parked outside Kassim's place.

'Is he in?' I called out to the boy in the shop before getting out.

'Yes,' he shouted back.

I was immediately shown to Kassim's office.

'What are you still doing here?' he exclaimed. 'I had expected you to have left. Almost everyone has gone.'

'You haven't!' I pointed out with a weak grin.

'No, but perhaps I'm stupid!'

'Then there are two of us!' I laughed too, feeling at home with him and somewhat protected by his attitude and the ambience of his cosy office.

'What can I do for you?' he asked, surprise still etched on his face.

I produced the white cloth from my left jeans pocket and placed it on the desk. It was the first time I'd looked inside and I was surprised by how many diamonds there were, of all shapes and sizes. He inspected each one while I drank my customary iced Coke.

'You have more than usual,' he nodded, looking up at me as though he expected a reaction or explanation.

'How much for all of these, Kassim? The market must be good with all the unrest.'

'Yes, people want small, portable valuables. I will give you three thousand American dollars.'

As before, I could neither argue nor negotiate: I had no knowledge about the value of rough diamonds. He counted out the dollars and, as he did so, I said: 'I have one more diamond for you today. My last diamond, in fact.'

I reached deep inside my right jeans pocket to find Scarlett's solitary diamond. Kassim stopped counting as I laid my prized offering on the black velvet square in front of him. As I released my hand he glanced at me and then studied the diamond. His first reaction was shock, and then, with growing excitement, he looked more closely through his lupe.

For a long while Kassim didn't speak. I resisted the urge to ask questions or comment. It was clear that the stone was exceptional; even with my scant education about gems I had not appreciated its size and brilliance. I waited and waited. Finally Kassim lifted his head and put down his magnifying glass.

'This is a very interesting diamond, Eric. Where does it originate from, and how did you come by it?'

Kassim had never questioned me before, but this diamond had aroused his curiosity.

'You like the diamond then,' I answered, avoiding the question but looking him straight in the eye.

'Yes I do, and I want to buy it from you. It is a very good size and, cut well, it could be very valuable.'

I appreciated his honesty and then volunteered: 'Does it matter where the stone comes from? This country is about to fall apart with little or no hope of surfacing to where it is today for many years. It is the last diamond I'll ever bring you, Kassim, so let's part with you having the diamond and me having the dollars.'

He knew that what I said was true. Prince Johnson had already passed the point where I had met up with the children and I would never go back there. That part of the bush was now out of reach to Kassim as well, although I kept the location to myself.

Would Kassim offer me enough to pay Gihad and to buy tickets for Sue and me as well? At that moment nothing mattered more. I just wanted to be out of the country before the ceiling fell in. I also realised that, by now, Scarlett and my other saviours could have been killed by the marauding prince.

I showed no emotion when Kassim said that he would give me $6,000 for Scarlett's diamond, and my mind flew straight to the little girl. She and the other children were about to buy my escape from one of Africa's bloodiest coups. I felt so grateful to them all.

Conflict diamonds are now commonly spoken of as a means of funding warring factions. In 1990 I was actually selling my diamond to escape the conflict! I thanked Kassim and left with $9,000 stuffed in my pocket: enough to pay Gihad's bribe and for our tickets.

Tempting as it was to go to a nearby cafe to have some time and space to mull matters over, I realised that I was far too conspicuous. I hadn't spotted another white face since leaving the house that morning. And, carrying so much cash, I was vulnerable to assault and robbery, as well as another possible arrest by any of the trigger-happy military men.

Back in the office I hid the money safely in the radio room and sat back to listen to the multi-coloured mynah birds. They reminded me of my childhood and listening to bird songs with my parents, though of course not in abject fear. I wondered where the years had gone and reflected that much of what I'd achieved had now been lost, and that just staying alive was now my main priority. I worried about Lavoisier and Siafa and all my other local staff, and what would happen to them; thankfully, I knew that my five European expatriate staff already had plans in place to leave.

In that moment I felt the loss of Scarlett and the children, as well as a profound regret that I would never be able to thank them for my freedom. How I wished I could repay them in some way.

It was time to call Gihad and tell him that I had the funds. He had provisionally booked two seats on the 9 p.m. flight on Friday, which was the last ever commercial plane leaving Liberia. However, he'd also told me that he wouldn't confirm the seats until I had paid for the tickets and confirmed that I had $8,000 for him.'

Knowing I had the money gave me an inner calm when I picked up the phone and asked him to come round – this was not a conversation to be having on the telephone.

He was soon inside my office. 'You could be lying about the $8,000.'

'If I am lying then you won't let Sue and me on the plane on Friday. I will give you the money when you take us to the plane and Sue is out of the car. When she is safe, you would still have me! I'm not stupid enough to stay in the country. You are the blackmailer, so you will understand why I don't trust you.'

Worded like that, he had no option but to agree.

'Okay, but I need the ticket money now and a bit extra for the travel agent to keep your name quiet, and for the customs and exit documents at the airport – say $1,500.'

'Where does this end?' I raged at Ghiada. 'That's it, nothing else, and get out of here.'

'I am taking a big risk too. All eyes are on you so I'm exposed by helping you,' he shouted back.

'You are a shareholder of this company too, and you know exactly what we do and that it's all legal.'

'Yes, but the government doesn't think so. It's only going to get worse and I'm leaving too, which is why I want the money. If I get out, you get out – but if not, you are here with me.'

It was an ugly stalemate. I paid him the $1,500 and was now short of $500, but that would be far easier to find. Our departure was just a few days away. I counted down every hour. I counted down every minute. All that mattered was our escape from Liberia.

I still woke and vomited every morning, and the creditors still hung around at the gates all day. There were certainly fewer of them now, although the remaining protesters were tenacious and vocal.

There was nothing I could do for them other than listen. I knew that Sue was not going to like the news of our departure and planned to tell her late on Friday afternoon. Otherwise I was certain that she would insist on doing a round of final farewells, which might jeopardise our arrangements.

Later that day Antonio Vasquez, our Spanish bush manager, arrived in town, en-route to leaving the country. He'd worked for me since I'd bought into Cape Palmas Logging and we'd become good friends. We had a coffee together in the office and he asked me what I was going to do. I told him my plans and explained how I was now $500 short.

'Don't worry,' he assured me. 'I'll loan you the money.'

I was so thrilled by his kindness, and in fact he lent me $700 so I had a bit extra for myself. He never asked any questions, but smiled and wished me well.

As Friday grew nearer, the longer the time seemed to stretch and my nerves felt even more strained. There were no further incidents with the government or military during those last few days. I prayed for Friday to come. The country was heading for lockdown, with no commercial planes or vessels arriving or departing. That last flight was my only hope.

By then the tension was really ratcheting up. The radio reported that Johnson was on the outskirts of Monrovia, just a few miles north of us in Sinkor, although it was hard to know how accurate the bulletins were. We relied on the BBC World Service each Sunday; they had no good news to offer. Stories filtered through of long queues at the border into Sierra Leone. Anyone with even a tenuous link to

Doe[13] or his regime was fleeing from the coming reprisals. Taxis, buses and lorries were piled high with people and their belongings. It was impossible to make an international call; receiving a call was a little better, but you'd generally be cut off unexpectedly during the conversation. I felt utterly alone with little support or advice from any quarter. The British Embassy had merely advised people to leave immediately, but offered no assistance with flights out.

Siafa remained stoic throughout. I asked him what he intended to do and he said that he was going to stay. He had survived coups before and knew what he needed to do. I didn't question him further.

Friday morning finally came and I decided what to take with me. I left most of my clothes and personal belongings behind. I crammed paperwork into my briefcase. The morning dragged slowly by until lunchtime when Lavoisier and Gihad arrived and we sat down with Siafa.

Our plan was that Gihad would arrive in a taxi, park near the house, then come in to collect Sue and me. He would accompany us and make all the arrangements at the terminal, before the taxi drove along the runway to the waiting plane, bound for Tenerife.

The four of us had coffee and we talked about how all our efforts had amounted to nothing in the face of the imminent coup. We spoke for quite a time before Lavoisier and Gihad had to leave. I said a private farewell to Lavoisier, hugging him as I held back my emotions. My office manager and friend shared Siafa's confidence of surviving the troubles.

I had an hour to wait before I planned to tell Sue. I strolled

---

13   During the 1980 Liberian coup, Master Sergeant Samuel Doe – backed by the CIA, who viewed Doe as a strategic cold war ally – overthrew and killed President William Tolbert. Doe ordered the execution of a majority of Tolbert's cabinet publicly and brutally on the beach near the Executive Mansion in front of a jubilant crowd and the world's press.

around the garden, immersing myself in the scents and colours of the flowers and birds for one last time. It was such a serene scene – such a contrast to the hell being unleashed just a few miles away.

The time had come to tell Sue all about our imminent departure. I took a few gulps of the scented air and, with my heart in my mouth, clutched her hand tightly.

'We're booked on a flight tonight at 9 o'clock to Tenerife. I know it's short notice, but we'll come back soon.'

My second statement was simply not true. There was no way anyone could return to an inferno of death and destruction.

Sue was clearly annoyed, most probably because she had so little time to get organised. I explained that we couldn't take much and that we were leaving by taxi at 6.30. By now she was furious and disappeared to say goodbye to her friends nearby, before returning to pack hastily. Then Gihad arrived on time and we had to go.

We said goodbye to Siafa, who hugged Sue and then nodded at me and wished us well. We also said our farewells to the gate boy and cook. Neither of them knew what we were doing. As we left I heard the familiar sound of the heavy gate-bolt locking into position for the final time.

Sue cried uncontrollably. 'I can't leave my dogs. Who will look after them?'

She gave a final hug to Buster, a Liberian street dog with a lovely temperament. Of course, Sue thought that she would be returning to her animals.

It was a long, intense drive to the airport, with Gihad clearly anxious, in the front, and Sue furious beside me, in the back. I was silent all the way. Thankfully, I had been spared further arrests that week, but we had several road blocks to cross before reaching the airport. Gihad calmly talked us through each roadblock.

My heart was beating quickly and I shook as sweat poured down my face. The taxi driver dropped Gihad off on the approach road to the airport and parked nearby without lights.

'Where's Gihad gone?' demanded Sue.

'To get the boarding passes,' I replied.

'Why are we waiting in the car? Why aren't we with him?'

'Please just trust me – we'll be on the flight shortly.'

It felt an age since Gihad left. I feared being seen and questioned about my movements. The whole country was on the brink of disaster and the main airport was a potential hotspot. The place was teeming with military personnel and vehicles. Finally Gihad returned and sat down in the front of the car.

'It's all sorted – let's drive on now,' he whispered, also shaking like a leaf.

He gave directions to the taxi driver. We approached the perimeter fence until we came to a small gap. This had been prepared for our dangerous mission. I decided not to mention this part of the plan to the ever inquisitive Sue. We drove through and could see the Iberia jet on the runway with the steps down at the back, ready to take off.

Whatever plans Gihad made, they were meticulous and running smoothly so far. All looked quiet as we approached the rear end of the plane. I winced with apprehension: moments away from freedom.

The engines were already running and the haze of fumes formed swirling clouds in the late evening air. A flight attendant had spotted the car and came down the steps to greet us. Gihad looked at me and handed over Sue's passport and boarding pass. Still in a state of confusion, she climbed out of the taxi and walked up the steps.

Then she stopped, halfway up, as I sat in the taxi and the plane's engines roared. She looked over at me, obviously wondering why I was still in the car. I beckoned her to continue and she disappeared from view.

I began to tremble. All the battles I'd fought, all my trials and tribulations, and all my escape plans, came down to this one moment. On the plane, I would live; left behind, I would die. My heart pounded, pounded and pounded even more.

I sighed with enormous relief as Sue disappeared inside the aircraft. At the same time the flight attendant, her skirt swirling in the fierce exhaust fumes, urged me to hurry up. I handed Gihad the envelope and said: 'Check it if you want.'

'There's no need; you didn't know I wouldn't, so I'm sure it's all there. Here's your passport and boarding pass. I apologise for putting you in this position, but I need money to get my family out.'

I shook his hand: 'I wish you well, my friend.'

The taxi turned around on the runway and made a speedy exit.

My heart was thumping as I approached the plane. I raced up the steps and, as soon as I reached the top, the stairway was automatically retracted. I expected the steps to go down again or the engines to stop; at any moment, I knew that one call to the pilot could put an end to my escape plan.

Dazed from it all, I sat down next to Sue with our one suitcase close to the back the plane. The urgency of our situation was brought home when I spotted Quinca and his wife further down the aisle. I noticed other familiar faces among the thirty or so people making their bids for freedom. I was sure that none of them had to organise such a dramatic series of events.

The screaming engines of the McDonnell Douglas MD-83, roaring to a crescendo, thrust the aircraft forward in this final, frenetic flight.

'Lift, lift,' I muttered, not knowing whether the flight would be aborted or the pilot was pushing everything to the limit.

'Lift, lift,' I hissed as the runway continued to flash past.

Within seconds the aircraft was lifting off the ground and I watched the distant lights of Monrovia come into sight as the plane rapidly gained height. I felt as free as those eagles, viewed from the airstrip at Port Greenville.

The relief was instant. My heart returned to normal with the realisation that we had escaped the chaos and terror of Liberia. I sat quietly in my seat as a wave of emotions swept over me.

I don't remember how long the flight was to Tenerife – it must have been three hours or so – but I recall Sue's rage when I delivered even more bad news.

'We're not coming back,' I admitted. 'We can't come back. It's going to get horrific in Liberia. It'll be a bloodbath, believe me.'

'I can't believe what you're telling me,' she fumed. 'You should have told me all this.'

'If I'd told you, then you would have been even more worried. I couldn't take the chance that it would leak out. We were lucky to get out in the end.'

Sue was bereft at the thought of never seeing her dogs again, particularly Buster, and dismayed at having left behind so many of her clothes – not to mention the goodbyes never said to friends. I tried to explain why I'd kept our departure so secret and why our escape had to be so low key. She wasn't in the mood for listening and the journey was fraught with her grief at leaving.

The night air was warm when we landed in Tenerife, and the change in atmosphere from conflict-stricken Liberia to the small sub-tropical holiday island was immense. I remember my surprise on our first morning when I didn't feel – and wasn't – physically sick. We tried to relax in what were calm, normal surroundings while waiting for seats on one of the many charter planes heading back to England. Throughout that time Sue remained unhappy with the decision which, she felt, I had thrust upon her. I felt sad about Sue's reaction, but I was just relieved that we had escaped with our lives.

It was summer and finding seats wasn't easy but, after fleeing just ahead of a coup, waiting three days for a flight was nothing to me. For us, things could only get better now. For Liberia, that was another matter.

Within days of our departure, Liberia's three-way civil war was raging, involving the different hordes led by Samuel Doe, Charles Taylor and Prince Johnson. While Taylor's guerrilla forces controlled much of the country, Johnson's insurgents had reached the streets of Monrovia. Despite attempts by the Economic Community of West African States to persuade Doe to resign and go into exile, he stood his ground and remained besieged in his mansion, guarded by Israeli-trained soldiers.

By early June four American warships arrived off the coast of Liberia. It was not until 6 August 1990 that US President Bush sent in over two hundred marines. They evacuated seventy-four Americans and foreign dependants who were trapped at the American Embassy in Monrovia.

After a bloody gun battle, Samuel Doe was seized by Johnson and his rebels on 9 September. He was tortured, mutilated and finally brutally murdered by Johnson and his mob. The whole gruesome spectacle was videotaped, edited and a soundtrack added. The barbaric affair was widely distributed by Johnson to news agencies who broadcast the disturbing events to horrified viewers around the world.

In this depraved home movie, Johnson is seen behind a massive desk with a garland of grenades around his neck, being fanned by a woman and drinking a can of beer. An interrogation of sorts is taking place as Johnson tries to extract information from Doe about where he has stashed money. Between Doe's screams and snippets of information about Swiss bank accounts, Johnson is barking orders at his drunken thugs to hack off Doe's body parts, bit by bit. Doe haemorrhaged to death later that night.

After Doe's death, the bloody civil war continued between Johnson's rebels and Charles Taylor's forces until 1996. The conflict was punctuated by seven failed peace conferences in various regional capitals, and a failed coalition government. Estimates of the death toll vary between 110,000 and 200,000, and it is considered one of Africa's bloodiest ever wars. In addition, a million Liberians were displaced into refugee camps in neighbouring countries, and entire villages were left empty after people fled at various times. Eventually peace negotiations and foreign involvement led to a ceasefire and Johnson fled into exile in Nigeria. Charles Taylor was elected President of Liberia in July 1997.

Liberians had voted for Taylor in the hope that the bloodshed would finally end, and while it did decrease considerably, it did not stop completely. Violent incidents occurred frequently after the end of the war, while Taylor spread an ever-increasing net of corruption across the country, reducing Liberia to a blighted backwater. The once viable economic infrastructure went into sharp decline.

Taylor was instrumental in promoting conflict in neighbouring Sierra Leone, where fifty thousand died. He was a ruthless profiteer and amassed a huge fortune in so-called blood diamonds.

The Second Liberian Civil War began in 1999 and lasted until 2003, when Taylor resigned as President and sought refuge from his opponents in Nigeria. In 2004, Prince Johnson returned to Liberia from his exile and resumed his political career; at the time of writing he is currently Senior Senator for Nimba County, in north-central Liberia.

In 2006, Taylor was arrested and taken to The Hague to stand trial in a special UN-backed court, the proceedings taking place in Holland to prevent renewed unrest in West

Africa. At the end of a four-year trial Taylor was found guilty on eleven charges including sexual slavery, looting of blood diamonds, terrorism, rape, murder and use of child soldiers by rebel groups during Sierra Leone's 1991-2002 conflict. The rebels were notorious for hacking off the limbs of civilians to terrorise the population.

Witnesses for the prosecution said that Taylor had armed the rebels in exchange for diamonds mined by slave labourers. During the trial it emerged that the model Naomi Campbell had controversially received diamonds from Charles Taylor after meeting him at an event in South Africa in 1997. Charles Taylor is the first former head of state to be convicted of war crimes since the Nuremberg Trials after World War Two; he was sentenced to fifty years in jail, which he is currently serving in the UK.

I found out later that all five of my European workers got out safely, which was a relief indeed. I have no idea what happened to Siafa Sherman, Lavoisier Tubman and the other local Cape Palmas Logging workers. Sadly, my attempts to contact them during and after the conflict amounted to nothing.

The same applies to Scarlett and the other children in the bush. I imagine that they suffered horribly at the hands of the rampaging rebels. I read that children were mutilated, raped and killed by the advancing brutes.

And yet Scarlett and her little chums saved my life. And how did I repay them for their precious diamonds?

A few bags of rice.

CHAPTER THIRTEEN

Back in England

August 4th 2014. Day thirteen at St George's Hospital.

The morning follows its regular routine. Late in the afternoon Dr Mickey Koh comes into my room to ask how I feel the procedure is going. I tell him how pleased I am with everything, and he confirms that the hospital is also very happy with my progress. He is optimistic that there will be white cells in my blood test this Friday. That will be a week after my transplant, which will be amazing. Of course, that lifts my already good mood even higher.

Axel emails me in the evening. He tells me that the bruising in his arms has gone, and all that remains from the stem cell harvest are the marks where the needles were inserted into his arms. As ever he is more concerned with my health than his own, and I'm touched yet again by his thoughtfulness. He also tells me that he has been informed by DKMS (the German Bone Marrow Donor Centre who work closely with Anthony Nolan) that he will be 'locked' on their register as my exclusive donor for the next two years. I feel fortunate and privileged.

August 5th 2014. Day fourteen St George's Hospital.

I'm feeling upbeat, apart from a headache caused by the anti-rejection drug Cyclosporine, and high blood pressure drugs. But overall, I'm in a positive mood. I have practised living within my surroundings and embracing all that I have to do here – and with books, puzzles, TV, iPod, iPad and iPhone there is a lot to keep me occupied. My daughters and brothers have been in touch every day. Although in an isolation room, I feel far from isolated.

All in all, I feel I've made the best use of my time here – although I still haven't looked out of the window to the outside world!

I remember the thrill of looking out of a plane window during that flight from Tenerife to Gatwick.

★★★

We spent three days trying to arrange a flight from Tenerife to England, and eventually secured a booking with Iberia.

I felt so fortunate to be with Sue, on another Iberia aircraft, heading for Gatwick. The fields and woodlands of Sussex filled me with emotion as I gazed out of the window and we prepared to land.

I felt overwhelming relief not only that we'd survived, but also that I would now be able to see Vicky and Louisa again. Sue, unaware of all that was happening in Liberia, didn't feel that same sense of reprieve.

We left Gatwick and then travelled up to Cumbria to stay with Sue's parents, Gordon and Jean, who I knew well.

I was given a superb welcome, even though there was a palpable distance between Sue and myself. We monitored the news bulletins in England. The tragedy really hit home when we heard about a massacre of six hundred refugees, soon after we left. The victims, mostly women and children, had sought sanctuary in St Peter's Lutheran Church not far from our house in Sinkor.

My decision to leave appeared to be justified, with all of those reports coming out, but our relationship continued to cool. I felt that she'd lost all respect for me – no doubt because I didn't actually tell her that we were leaving Liberia for ever.

From Cumbria I made several trips on my own to see Vicky and Louisa, who were now twenty and eighteen respectively and starting university.

I told Sue that I had to return to Jersey to deal with the financial chaos, caused by the coup. She had no desire to return to the island. I simply accepted her decision and spent a couple of days in Great Yarmouth with my younger brother David, en-route to Jersey. The sights and sounds had not changed since my first job there as a shipping clerk.

None of my family had any idea of what I'd been through in Africa, although I discussed some of the details with David. It was great to see him and comforting for me to stay with family while I was feeling rather sorry for myself.

Sleep was a struggle. On my second morning in Great Yarmouth I woke up early and took a slow walk along the promenade. A chill breeze came in off the North Sea, but the summer sun would soon rise and warm the air. I saw a beach cafe open up and I became their first customer of the day. I enjoyed a mug of tea as the waves crashed over the sand.

My mind wandered between thoughts of heading to Jersey and the fact that Sue wanted to stay in Cumbria. As I continued to take in the familiar surroundings, I received a loud and clear wake-up call...

My gaze was drawn to a people carrier. Slowly six paraplegics, strapped into wheelchairs, were taken down the vehicle's ramp and brought into the cafe by their helpers. I immediately realised that I had so much to be grateful for – my health, my daughters and family, and felt ashamed that I was so miserable.

In that moment, I vowed never to submit to self-pity in the face of personal trauma. I walked back to David's house with lifted spirits and told him the story. The next day I left Norwich Airport, bound for Jersey...but without Sue.

I arrived on the island at lunchtime and headed straight

for my apartment in St Helier. Again, the surroundings hadn't changed; the only difference was in my financial situation. I'd run out of cash and my credit cards were almost up to their limit. I was also aware that it would probably take me several months to sort out my business affairs on the island. I was unsure of what, if anything, I would have left at the end of it all. My thoughts turned to Scarlett and her wisdom in knowing that there's little point in having assets if you don't have any food.

I summoned my courage and made appointments at the two banks where I had outstanding – and substantial – loans. One bank had loaned money to Cape Palmas Logging, and the other held the mortgage on my apartment.

I was anxious and uncertain about the possible outcomes, but ready to face up to my responsibilities and deal with the consequences, whatever they might be.

At the first bank, I was utterly astonished by the manager's reaction. He told me that he had been following the dramatic news about Liberia and was relieved that I had escaped the conflict. He said that, under the circumstances, there was little that the bank could do and he was certain that it would write off the debt. Of course this was not the reaction I'd been expecting, and it certainly relieved the pressure. It is true that, 90% of the time, whatever you fear in a situation does not materialise.

The second bank manager, where I held my mortgage, had also been watching the news. He said he was glad that I had made it out of Liberia but they required the loan to be repaid or kept up to date. My only way out of that was to sell the apartment, and again luck was on my side as another resident in the block wanted to buy the place.

We settled on a price to include the contents. After the mortgage, credit cards and overdraft were paid off I was left with my clothes and a few personal effects, plus enough money to keep me going for a year or so. I was fine with that; I had my life and a new perspective. What I wanted more than anything at that point was to rest and recuperate.

My affairs took until the end of 1990 to sort out. Despite all the previous traumas, I could now take my life in any direction. I nevertheless had moments of despondency and loneliness where I had no idea what to do next, and really felt weighed down by the loss of Sue, my home and my business.

Florida beckoned, and a holiday with friends Anita and Victor. I'd known them since my Scottish experiences. They were the Edinburgh dealers for my favourite Aston Martin cars.

I'd always enjoyed being in Florida and loved the people, the place and the weather. I was in no rush to leave, save to see my family and a handful of friends.

After a few weeks I returned to Aberdeen to spend some time with Vicky and Louisa and then travelled down to Cumbria to see Sue. Unfortunately, the distance between us had only grown and I realised that our relationship was, without doubt, beyond repair. I desperately wanted her back, but the atmosphere told me there was no hope.

Back in Florida, with Anita and Victor, I enjoyed sightseeing in Orlando. I had enough cash to pay the deposit on two houses; I rented one out and lived in the other.

Network marketing was taking off at the time, and I liked the American 'team building' ideas. I promoted a company and their products very successfully. I even had an office in downtown Orlando and drove around in a large grey four-door Cadillac Brougham.

I was absolutely stunned by the size of Orlando. There were seven nightclubs in Disney World. They were housed in Pleasure Island; the idea was that one payment would ensure admission to all of the clubs. New Years' Eve fireworks parties were held every night.

With the great Florida climate, wonderful food and friendly people, and trips to Disney when family and friends were visiting from England, I felt that I was permanently on holiday. I could come and go when I liked, work as and when I wanted, and I was content with my life.

After five years of living the American dream, I woke up and decided that the lure of my home country was pulling me back...

By 1996 I was living in London in the Old Brompton Road, renting a flat on the top floor of a building with a nightclub in the basement. It was time to put roots down again and, having sold one of the houses in Kissimmee, I bought a house in Bracknell, to the southwest of London.

Not long after moving in, I received a call from my brother David. He told me that our father had developed a chest infection and been admitted to hospital. At once, Gary and I travelled up to Great Yarmouth. He looked frail and old in the hospital bed. I reflected on how he'd looked when we'd all lived together as a family, which didn't seem that long before, and now here he was – elderly and fragile.

He'd been through numerous health scares before and I wondered if this was yet another one that he'd come through. Aged fifty-two he'd had a massive heart attack. He was not expected to survive, but he proved the doctors wrong with true Evans tenacity and even returned to work.

However, during his early sixties he started to show signs of a change in his personality, and in the space of a year he lost the ability to walk normally. This was so sudden and dramatic that Gary arranged for him to be seen by a neurologist in London. He had lost the memory area for walking as part of a long-standing process of blockage of tiny blood vessels.

The slow but relentless loss of his brain tissue, resulting from this process, had left him clinically demented. A CT scan soon confirmed that large areas of his brain had been destroyed by microscopic clots. The tiny clots had come from the scar tissue of his damaged heart muscle, ever since his heart attack. By his late sixties he was unable to look after himself and eventually moved into a care home, where he appeared to be happy enough.

As we sat with Dad in the hospital, I wondered what he was thinking and feeling as he looked at his three sons. He knew he was so ill that he could die at any moment. The four of us talked about the best of old times, including the tortuous car journeys and our seaside holidays.

After a few days Gary and I returned to London with the promise that we'd come back to visit him on his birthday in a few days' time. On the morning of his seventy-second birthday, 28 December 1998. David received a call from the hospital saying that our father had succumbed to the bronchopneumonia and died peacefully in his sleep.

It was a shock, even though we knew the moment was coming. I was grateful that he had died in his sleep and that I was with my brothers when I heard the news. It seemed somehow profound that it had happened on his birthday; as if the circle of his life was complete.

I spent New Year in Great Yarmouth with David, his partner Jeanette and some of their friends. We had muted New Year celebrations as we prepared for Dad's funeral during the first week in January.

The bleak weather matched our mood. Only around twenty people attended; the short and simple service appeared to mirror his life.

After the funeral Gary, David and I strolled along the seafront and shared our memories over fish and chips in one of the promenade restaurants. After our meal, we had a few drinks in town and fondly reminisced about Mum and Dad.

I was forty-six and wondered what would be happening in my life a year into the future.

Little did I know that events in January would have a profound effect, not only on the year ahead, but on the rest of my life.

CHAPTER FOURTEEN

My World Imploded

August 6th 2014. Day fifteen at St George's Hospital

I'm really starting to feel much better, especially as the doctors are now giving me two codeine painkillers before each dose of Cyclosporine. I'm taking the rejection drug daily because of severe headaches.

I compare my recent transplant with the procedure in 2004. I realise that I have not been sick once this time, and I assume that must demonstrate the progress made in medicine over the past ten years.

Between the routine check-ups from medical staff and my meals, I spend the day quietly, absorbed in my books, puzzles and all the entertainment at my disposal. Later on I either Face Time or text my various family members, and then go to sleep, feeling comfortable and calm.

★★★

A short time after my father's funeral Jeff, an American marketing colleague, helped me out with a few business issues.

'What can I do to repay you both?' I asked his wife.

'You don't look 100%; promise me that you'll make an appointment and visit your doctor,' she said.

I kept my promise and the doctor duly took a blood sample. He phoned the next day with the results.

'Sit down immediately and do not walk after this call. Arrange for someone to take you to Wexham Park Hospital as soon as possible, and ask them to get a wheelchair for you from reception.'

Clearly thinking they had my results mixed up with someone else as I was feeling fine, I jumped in my car and drove to the hospital. At reception I gave my name and asked for directions.

'How did you get here?' the receptionist asked, studying my notes on her computer.

'I drove,' I answered, unsure of what all the fuss was about.

'Take a seat now, and the doctor will see you soon.'

Minutes later a tall, white-coated doctor ushered me into a consulting room.

'You shouldn't be able to walk,' he began. 'Your haemoglobin (Hb) concentration is 5 when it should be between 14–16, and your platelet count is so low that if you cut yourself it will be difficult to stop the blood.'

He said that, to get to the root of the problem, he would have to take a sample of bone marrow and bone from inside my leg. We would then know whether I was suffering from a serious lack of vitamins and minerals, myelofibrosis, or leukaemia. He also said that he would give me a blood transfusion of three units of blood and keep me in for various tests.

So within an hour of my doctor's phone call, I was in a hospital gown, on a ward about to receive three units of blood. More than anything I felt shock, and also some annoyance at the disruption to my work plans for that week.

The following morning the oncologist confirmed that I had myelofibrosis. He went on to explain that I would require regular blood transfusions. But he could not predict how much or how often, and at some point I would also require a bone marrow transplant. I was certainly not in good shape.

I felt my world imploding over the next few days while I came to terms with my condition and how it might affect my future. The outlook was not good. The oncologist had explained the process of finding a bone marrow donor, and the radiotherapy and chemotherapy required. My life expectancy was limited. I decided to explore alternative therapies and hopefully cure myself.

Within a few days I left the hospital and went home to contemplate on the changes needed in my new life. I started juicing fruit and vegetables every day, slept a great deal and began meditating. My mind was now set to be positive and remain as healthy as I could while I researched different treatments. Although I was attending Wexham Park Hospital regularly for various tests, it soon became clear that I would need a transfusion of two to three units of blood every six weeks.

My brother Gary showed his practical side. 'If you die, where would you like to be buried?'

'I want to be cremated,' I replied, 'and my ashes scattered at the top of Scafell Pike in the Lake District.'

I had climbed to the summit at the age of ten and again at forty. I chose the magnificent landscape for my final resting place, in the event of my death.

A friend of mine, Susan, who lived in Henley, suggested that I should visit two women who administered Reiki from a house nearby. I made an appointment. The house was an imposing brick and flint mansion. I was asked to wait in the hall.

A few minutes later an affable woman introduced herself as Vickie and led me to a room on the first floor where I met her twin sister, Jacky. The treatment – administered by both ladies – was relaxing and I felt comfortable with the two sisters.

We soon became good friends and, during one appointment, I could hear piano music. How good was that? I thought to myself that the pianist should be on stage. What a sound.

The music stopped and the door to the treatment room opened. In stepped Vickie's husband, Jon Lord of Deep Purple. All I needed at that moment was for Ritchie Blackmore to walk in, play a few chords and complete my day.

'Hi, nice to meet you,' Jon grinned, not really needing any introduction, with his distinctive grey hair tied back as usual.

'Brilliant to meet you,' I replied enthusiastically.

I felt like the equivalent of a 'soldier of fortune' as I shook his hand – and learned that Jacky was married to Ian Paice, Deep Purple's drummer.

Over the forthcoming months I was invited to various meetings for alternative therapies at their house, and Vickie gave me huge amounts of support during that time.

As the millennium approached a German friend in Marbella, Udo, with whom I'd been marketing vitamin and mineral products, suggested that I come down and spend some time there. Since we were already working together and I knew the area well, I didn't need to think too long before taking him up on the offer.

Soon I'd put my house in Berkshire on the market and was installed in an apartment at the Aloha Gardens, a mile into the mountains, close to Puerto Banus. A large balcony overlooked beautiful, colourful gardens with a stunning backdrop.

I continued working with Udo, using his office in the port to market health products into Germany and the UK. Just being there was idyllic and relaxing as I loved the mountains, beaches, harbour views and sunshine. I kept up my regime of relaxing, juicing and meditation, and began to search for alternative cures.

Fortunately that part of Spain has a multitude of alternative practitioners and I began by meeting a doctor in St Pedro, not far from Marbella, who put electrodes on my head and tested my brain function – thankfully no problems were detected.

Then I heard about Dr. Ravi Ponniah, an iridologist in Islington, London, who offered a variety of treatments. I tried a detoxifying footbath where my feet were immersed in saltwater and an electric current was passed through to draw out toxins. It appeared to work as the water turned dark, and I felt much better afterwards.

After that came light therapy, when Ravi played music as I watched varying coloured lights flash through glasses on my head. Later, he injected Ozone (O3) into my body. Before he began the treatment, he showed me a small amount of my dark red blood. It turned bright red when he injected the ozone.

Ravi and I became good friends, and I had further ozone treatments from him while I stayed at a beautiful house in Santa Fe, New Mexico. This is the oldest state capital in America and also the highest, at over 7,000 feet above sea level. The sunsets were spectacular every evening, colouring surrounding mountains orange and purple. I was there for a week and, aside from my treatments, enjoyed sightseeing in and around the city. On my return to Europe I experienced the longest gap I ever had between blood transfusions. Tranquillity and altitude must have been the keys to my improving health.

I stayed in Marbella for around a year between trips to the UK for blood transfusions and to visit my family, who also came out to Spain. The beaches and mountains were spectacular; simply wandering around Puerto Banus was an enjoyable pastime. The port is relatively new, having been built in 1970 by local property developer Jose Banus. It was the first ever port to be designed by a single architect, Russian Noldi Schreck, who styled it all like a sophisticated Andalusian village. There are bars, restaurants, nightclubs and elegant, branded shops. The marina there has become an iconic tourist destination with nearly five million visiting annually, including international celebrities and the super-rich, who descend with their exotic cars and luxury yachts.

I spent Christmas 2000 with one of my friends, Andreas Leopold, an ebullient character who lived beside Lake Zug in Switzerland in the winter and Marbella during the summer months. He was a few years younger than me and, on the surface, wild and brash. His clothes and cars were a perfect match. He drove a Ferrari, a Bentley and a Lamborghini. His clothes and cars were a perfect combination.

Andreas was also a speedboat enthusiast. His mean machine could outrun the local police boats and they tried to keep him on dry land.

When we visited Olivia Valere, the iconic nightclub near Marbella, a table beside the dance floor was cleared and several ice buckets with Crystal Champagne arrived for his guests. I really liked Andreas, and we occasionally spent quiet evenings together when I saw his softer side. Years later I was checking into the Hotel Hermitage in Monte Carlo, when Andreas walked in wearing a floor-length white fur coat and holding a tiny dog on a lead. His wife was dressed from head to toe in bright pink. He was an extraordinary character,

By the time I'd been living in Aloha Gardens for almost a year I needed to return to the UK more regularly for blood transfusions, because the myelofibrosis had progressed. My red blood cells, as always, were diminishing. This impacted on my iron levels because the body does not secrete the iron it receives from transfusions. To reduce those iron levels I had to use a special type of powered syringe, pumping the required solution into my stomach for twelve hours a day.

A friend in Marbella, who lived in Jersey, invited me to stay in St Helier. I discovered that little had changed in the Channel Islands. I soon slipped back into my old life there, as if I'd never been away. The main difference was that I visited the General Hospital in St Helier regularly to receive blood transfusions. A senior nurse, Maggs, went out of her way to look after me during those visits. I also made occasional trips to the Ruth Myles Unit at St George's Hospital as they specialised in bone marrow disorders including myelofibrosis.

That September, my family's lives took a serious turn when Vicky and Louisa's mum, Frances, lost her battle to cancer. Naturally, my daughters were devastated so I suggested that we do something together to celebrate her life. I made arrangements for the three of us, as well as Louisa's boyfriend Keith, to visit Marbella for a few days. There, we had ample time to pause and reflect.

On a lighter note I pursued a business venture, promoting health products with my good friend David Rondel who lived in Jersey. We travelled to Paris where we planned to tell other business people about our revolutionary ideas.

One of the assembled gathering proved to be a surprise package. A large, loud, bleached blonde lady named Chantal joined us for dinner. She placed a napkin over her cleavage to collect any spillage and ate with gusto. She consumed pigs' trotters, tripe and other horrendous looking side dishes as if her life depended on it.

Fat, grease and wine flew in all directions. I couldn't bear to watch as she sucked every last bone and splattered everyone on the table with debris. I took cover as the final remnants of her pig sucking orgy whistled past my ear. I could see that her interest in my health products was limited. She left the table, dripping with fatty residues, and still chewing on the tougher morsels. I have never seen a performance like that, anywhere on the planet, performed by man, woman or beast.

Her parting words filled me with dread: 'If you feel lonely tonight, my hotel door will be open.'

I politely declined, and whispered to David that perhaps he should consider the offer. We both waited until she disappeared in the lift and ran for our lives.

For my fiftieth birthday I returned to Marbella with close family and friends. I remember eating wonderful food in Toni Dalli's restaurant and gazing over the Mediterranean, wondering what lay in store during the next decade.

After living back in Jersey for several months, I could see countless opportunities in the booming property market on the island. Through a friend I was offered a job in an estate agents' office where I got to know the builders, developers and price of property.

I enjoyed the work and within a short time had become acquainted with many of the key people in the industry, at which point I set up my own property business. One of these developers asked me to remove all the agent's boards from a block of apartments on the beach in St Clements – and use my marketing skills. This was easier said than done as the planning department held that the block had been built in the wrong position, too close to the sea wall. The case was due to be argued in the local court and, in the interim, it was impossible to sell any of the properties. It was a case of so-called 'contingent liability'.

I decided to fix a selling price for each apartment and then offer them to buyers for 5% of that amount. That would serve as rent until title on the property was cleared and the fine, if any, was paid. On that basis the apartments were all soon snapped up by the people who were renting them. The developer paid the fine of £65,000 and everyone lived in the flats happily ever after.

David was, of course, extremely pleased with the outcome, and at that point I became his property problem fixer. His next request was, he said, an 'impossible one to sort out'.

<23966491136001505>

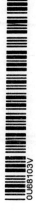

0U68103V

HIGHLAND BRIDGE CLUB
FAO: MR DANIEL SUTHERLAND
88 LAGGAN ROAD
INVERNESS
INVERNESS SHIRE
IV2 4EP

TNT 65

'This will show how good you really are,' he added. 'No one's been able to fix this – not even me.'

The problem revolved around another apartment block he owned and wanted to sell, this time in St Helier; and again he did not have clear title. When the block was built, one of its walls blocked a window in a nearby warehouse. No provision had been made with the owner of this building, so there was another issue of 'contingent liability'.

'I'll resolve it before the year's out,' I said, soaking up the summer sun.

He smiled and said nothing.

David's block of apartments had been built ten years earlier, but the building was dilapidated, having been poorly maintained. As a result, he was receiving low rents. I said that if I established clear title on the building then I would buy the whole block for £750,000 (knowing that I'd have to spend at least £150,000 on completely refurbishing all the apartments) and he agreed to the deal.

My problem was to find the principal of the warehouse whose window had been blocked. The building was owned by various family members who had inherited the warehouse, some of whom were under eighteen. Previously, they had been offered derisory compensation through lawyers: I decided to try a different approach.

I knew the people who rented the warehouse next door and they put me in touch with the daughter of the principal of the family. I met the woman and said I would like to meet her mother to discuss the warehouse and window issues. She explained that her mother lived on the mainland and seldom visited the island. She added that, having been approached before, the family was happy to leave matters as they were. I replied that I was so interested in talking with her that I would pay for her ticket to come over, because I had a serious proposition to make in person. She said she would tell her mother, but didn't think it would make the slightest difference.

I felt that if my 'different' message was conveyed, then it might strike a chord with the mother. Happily, my ploy worked. The daughter said her mother would see me for a few minutes during her next trip. Great, I thought; now I just have to make a good impression.

Some weeks later arrangements were made to meet the infamous mother at the apartments at 11 a.m. on a Sunday. I arrived early and heard a knock at the door. A tiny woman walked in with her husband and daughter. She strutted over towards me.

'What do you want?' she snapped, oozing authority from her mere four foot six frame.

'Well, I…' I tried to answer.

'Go on,' she rasped.

'Well I bought the building but I can't sell any of the flats without your approval.'

'That wasn't very clever,' she mocked. 'Maybe this should all have been checked out beforehand?'

I made my move. 'I realise that now. However, I only have £25,000 to assist you in helping with my problem.'

'If I was interested, then £25,000 is too small an amount to consider.'

'It's all I have,' I pleaded.

'Too bad then.'

How could I break the ice? I was facing a small lady with an enormous ego and possibly a large chip on her tiny shoulders. She had an attitude problem, and it was directed at me. She held all the aces in the pack, but it was time to play my joker.

Like a prince proposing to his princess, I got down on one knee and begged: 'Please sort out this matter for me. I implore you.'

The ice was broken. My nemesis suddenly exploded into laughter, showing a side to her character that had remained completely hidden. I knew that the price would go up, but the deal was on.

We negotiated over the next few days while details of the case became clear. There were seven family members, including children, who owned the warehouse, and only two among them lived in Jersey. Since all seven owners would have to appear before the court to complete the transaction, cost was her negotiating tool. By the middle of December we'd agreed on a figure of £50,000, which was actually less than I had feared. The local court set a date in early January for all seven family members to convene and complete the legal requirements.

The case duly went through on the appointed date and that afternoon I went to see David.

'You asked me to solve a problem for you and I have to tell you that I was not able to solve it within the period I set,' I said. 'However, it is now complete today, the 5th of January.'

David looked at me in disbelief.

And so, with the miniature mum happy, I bought the apartments for an increased price of £1 million. I refurbished the properties, and sold them on – at a profit of £500,000. I saw it as a unique window on the world of finance.

'I wish I'd known you fifteen years ago,' David said. 'Just think of all the problems you could have solved.'

From that moment on, all of David's tricky issues were diverted in my direction.

Around this time, I was invited to stay with Louisa and Keith at his family's holiday home on the beach in Rhosneigr, North Wales. Shortly afterwards I received a call from Louisa who told me that she had just accepted Keith's proposal for marriage.

I was thrilled for them both, and the following September they were married at Fasque House, a handsome baronial hall set in an exquisite country estate just south of Aberdeen. The magnificent building was the former home of Prime Minister William Gladstone in the early 1800s.

Louisa looked absolutely stunning. She is naturally beautiful with a wonderful warm smile, and on that day she was simply radiant, happy, calm and serene all at the same time. The dress, from Bridal Rogue Gallery in Chiltern Street, London, was fabulous and elegant. Giving Louisa away to Keith, who I knew would make a great husband for her, was a highlight of my life. It was such an honour to make a speech on Louisa's special day.

The following year I applied to the States of Jersey under the hardship rule to get my residency back. My application was supported by a letter from my doctor, detailing my daily medication. I was delighted when the States replied with a unanimous 'yes', adding that their review of my case had taken into account my contributions to the island's economy.

Obtaining my residency once more was fantastic news. It meant that I was able to move into my apartment on the beach at St Clement. As soon as the tenancy ended I moved in, refurbished the apartment, and finally made myself at home again.

Towards the end of 2003, the doctors at St George's made it clear that the transplant could no longer be postponed. My personal search for a cure had served the purpose of delaying that moment. On the medical front, since my initial diagnosis, a great deal of progress had been made in the treatment of my condition. If I'd had the procedure in 1996, then the heavy chemotherapy and radiography in use at the time would have given me a limited life expectancy.

In early 2004, Anthony Nolan confirmed that they had found a bone marrow match for me. This was an American man of fifty-three; I was told no more because of client confidentiality. In March I travelled to London where I stayed with my brother Gary while having preliminary tests at St

George's Hospital. Those duly over, I was admitted into the isolation unit and had a Hickman Line inserted, ready to begin chemotherapy the following day.

By morning, I was mentally and emotionally prepared for the procedure to begin. Five women, who had all been dealing with my care, entered my isolation room. They all looked sombre and the most senior, Dr. Judith Marsh, spoke first.

'There's no easy way to tell you this,' she said. 'Your donor has become unavailable and will not be able to give a bone marrow donation.'

I was politely told that there was nothing more the hospital could do for me at that point, and asked me to leave. That felt harsh, but it was a reality check. The isolation room would be needed for another patient with a match and ready to have a bone marrow transplant. However, they assured me that the search for a bone marrow donor would continue,

They soon left the room and, as the door closed behind them, I felt full of emotion. I could scarcely believe that I was so close, yet so far, from my transplant. I hurriedly packed then retreated to Gary's house, all the while trying to remain stoic.

I was reminded of my continuing belief: in the moment of something that seems so awful, there are the seeds of something good. However, will you recognise that feeling, and act upon it?

Although I didn't know of the event or timeline, I sincerely and completely believed that the story was far from over and something positive would come out of all this.

In the meantime, without the certainly of that knowledge, I returned to Jersey and my medical routine and business. But my body was struggling with the constant demand for blood transfusions – I required four units of blood every three weeks – and as a consequence there was the daily requirement of injections to reduce the iron overload. The situation could not continue for much longer.

A welcome boost to my spirits came in June when Jeanette, David's partner, gave birth to a daughter. It was a huge honour when they named their little girl Sydney, after my middle name.

I continued to believe that, despite the bad news about the American donor, the seeds of a positive outcome would grow and flourish. As I lay on the beach in Jersey, enjoying the last rays of the late summer sun, my mobile phone rang.

'Hi, it's Laura,' a friendly voice said.

My ears pricked up, because I knew I was talking to Laura, the transplant coordinator from the Ruth Myles Unit at St George's Hospital. What did she have to tell me?

'A donor has been found for you,' she told me, failing to hide the excitement in her voice.

'That is fantastic news,' I blurted out. 'Wonderful.'

I was ecstatic. Soon enough I had passed all the medical tests. Next, came an interview with the hospital psychologist.

'How are you going to cope with all this?' the psychologist asked. 'The Nurses will be coming in to give you treatment every four hours, whether you are asleep or not.'

'I feel very lucky to be in a situation where I have a donor and a team of people dedicated to keeping me alive. I'll do as they say – happily.'

I was admitted into room 3 in the isolation unit in September, barely a week after Laura's call.

Six days of chemotherapy followed. I had a rest day, then the bone marrow transplant. The entire procedure took thirty-three days. I left the hospital fifteen kilos lighter, in a wheelchair, bald and weak – but packed with optimism. My unknown young donor had provided me with millions of bone marrow cells. I was thrilled to be alive.

Throughout the bone marrow transplant my brother Gary was a staunch supporter, visiting me almost daily, and then afterwards nursing me back to health at his home in Peckham.

I stayed with him for two weeks and then, determined as ever to be strong, returned to Jersey and work.

I was also keen to contact my donor, who I knew to be young, male and German, to thank him for saving my life. I was told by Anthony Nolan that confidentiality would have to be preserved on both sides for two years. However, I was given permission to write a letter which Anthony Nolan would review and then forward. So I wrote my first letter of thanks and then a short while later received a response, with a few details crossed out to protect my donor's anonymity. We kept up our communication with letters to each other every few months.

In May 2005, for my brother David's fiftieth birthday, we all decided to celebrate the occasion in Monaco.

As a surprise I arranged for David and Jeanette to be taken from the airport to the hotel by helicopter to enjoy the aerial view of the coastline. Louisa, Keith and Gary, Vicky and I travelled there by taxi. In Monte Carlo we encountered my old friend Alan Murphy, the paper mill magnate. He invited us all for drinks on his 150-foot yacht, La Naturalle Dee.

And so on David's birthday we had lunch at a restaurant just down from the Café de Paris. After that we met Alan and his wife Wendy for drinks at The American Bar in the Hotel de Paris on the famous Place du Casino, before walking down with them both to their yacht.

We were given a tour of the fabulous vessel and then served drinks on deck, which gave us the perfect vantage point to enjoy the harbour spectacle in the warm spring sunshine. Late in the afternoon we went back to change at our hotel and then returned to the Hotel de Paris, where we ate at Le Grill, the restaurant on the top floor of the iconic hotel.

Not only was the food superb, but the views were breathtaking, as the restaurant overlooks the city and harbour, and also has a roof that slides back to reveal the night sky. It was a wonderful few days, which created special memories for us all.

That December, Gary and I flew out to Houston to spend a few weeks over Christmas with Louisa and Keith. Keith worked there as a geologist in the oil industry. Vicky travelled there separately from Scotland where she worked for the Turnberry Golf Club in Ayr. Gary had recently retired as an Ear, Nose and Throat surgeon, so he had time to go sightseeing with me. I revisited The Galleria, which I had last seen on my trip to the city thirty-three years before, when I was twenty-three and working for Hamilton Oil and Gas.

The vast mall had certainly stood the test of time and nothing much had really changed. There was still a multitude of stylish shops and restaurants and the hotel, where I had stayed all those years ago, and seeing everything again made me feel quite nostalgic. Nevertheless, it was tremendous to be back in Texas and we all spent a wonderful Christmas together. I was so proud to spend precious time with my daughters.

In September 2006, the two-year period of anonymity between my donor and me was finally up. Exactly two years to the day after my bone marrow transplant I contacted the Anthony Nolan Trust and was given my donor's name, Axel Drewes, and his address in Germany.

I wrote to him immediately, sending him a belated wedding present of a visit to The Residenz Heinz Winkler, a renowned Relais & Chateau Hotel and restaurant set in the mountains between Munich and Austria.

I couldn't wait to meet my saviour and his wife, so I invited them to spend a week's holiday with me in Spain the following spring. My German friends, Udo and Karen, joined me at Malaga Airport to help with translation.

We watched hundreds of people stream past before I

recognised tall and slim Axel and his wife from their wedding photo. As a surprise I'd hired a limousine to take him to the hotel in Marbella. What a feeling to be beside the man who had saved my life. He now called me his genetic twin!

We all spent a unique week together, eating out most evenings. We relaxed on the beach during the day, watching Axel playing football with Udo's two sons.

Our friendship really cemented. The week passed quickly, and towards the end I gave Axel a letter from Louisa:

Dear Axel,

I hope that you and Stephanie are enjoying your trip to Marbella and having lots of fun with my dad and everyone there. I'm really disappointed that Keith and I could not be there to join in the celebrations, but hopefully we will meet one day soon.

I just wanted to write a short note to thank you, but the words seem very small in comparison to the huge gift you have given my dad.

How do you thank the man who saved your dad's life? What are the words that fully explain the magnitude of your generosity and the selflessness of your actions?

What are the words that explain my gratitude to you, for my memories with him and that, without your generous nature, would be only a dream?

How do I thank you for making it possible for my dad to be here to look into the eyes of his grandchildren when they are born later this year?

There are no words.

With love to you both,

Louisa.

The correspondence continued when Axel and Stephanie left for the airport. Axel gave me a card, containing a prayer.

He told me: 'This card will take good care of you. And if you ever need anything else from me, know that you have it.'

Needless to say, my eyes clouded when I waved them goodbye. I still have the card in my wallet today.

That evening, during a solitary walk along the beach in Marbella, I reflected on my life and the importance of Axel's selfless actions. The full moon threw its light across the water, tracking me as I walked and surrounding me with a warm, happy glow.

I thought: Axel is truly a remarkable man: humble, generous, kind and thoughtful, and I am blessed to have his steadfast support.

Another invaluable friend, Chris Brien, came into my life around then when we were seated opposite each other at a dinner in Jersey. He was developing property on the island at the time and, like Axel, Chris has been unstinting in his support of me.

I invited Axel and Stephanie to Jersey for the annual International Air Display. How ironic: a German who had recently saved my life, watching aircraft that had bombed his country during the Second World War. And, of course, his predecessors had occupied the Channel Islands.

A few days after Axel and Stephanie's departure, on 14 September 2007, Louisa and Keith's twin daughters were born in Houston. They were seven weeks early, which is not uncommon for twins, and needed to spend some time in the Neonatal Intensive Care Unit (NICU) before they went home.

Thankfully they were both fairly healthy, but nevertheless they needed specialist neonatal care which was, of course, worrying for all concerned. I made plans to fly out to visit them a couple of weeks later and, after Louisa picked me up at the airport, I was taken back to their home in Houston.

A surprise awaited me. Beautiful Megan was fast asleep in

the double buggy. Louisa picked her out of the pram and then gave her to me. After all that Louisa had been through, I felt overwhelmed. Here was a perfect daughter for my daughter, who looked so happy and proud. I felt emotional as I held my granddaughter for the first time. A feeling of complete contentment came over me as well as the desire to just sit with Megan, and watch her face and delicate movements – just as I had with Louisa when she was born.

Isla was still in hospital, overcoming some feeding issues and had also suffered from Apnea of Prematurity. This condition means that infants stop breathing for twelve to twenty seconds during sleep, so we all visited her the following day.

My daughter Louisa describes the family's traumatic experience:

"Isla and Megan arrived on 14 September 2007. It had been a long and difficult journey to get that far but the physical and emotional roller-coaster finally paid off. Little did Keith and I know that we were about to get right back onto another one.

"They were seven weeks early, unexpected twins, and we knew that they would need one or perhaps two weeks in NICU before they could come home.

"They were both fairly healthy, Isla 4lb 13oz and Megan 4lb 7 oz. Megan needed a bit of help first with an IV line of caffeine. It was in her head, just above her forehead, which was very scary at first, but within a few days she was fine. Soon they both moved into the same cot together on the NICU ward.

"After a couple of days Isla started to have some feeding issues and had to have a feeding tube inserted through their nose. It looked terrible, but we knew this was the best way to get all the nutrients she needed directly into her tiny body. She was also suffering from Apnea of Prematurity; sometimes she would forget to breathe.

"Megan came home first, on 26 September 2007. It was seven years to the day after my mum passed away. Leaving the hospital was very difficult. We were overjoyed to be taking Megan home but devastated to leave Isla behind. It just felt wrong although we knew she was in the best possible place.

"The same day my dad was flying in from the UK and we decided to keep Megan's homecoming a surprise. I distinctly remember the moment he arrived and we showed him the big double buggy where Megan was sleeping.

"There are no words to describe that moment but there we were: Dad, Megan and me. After everything that we had all been through, he was about to hold one of his granddaughters for the first time. Dad met Isla in hospital the next day. He helped to feed her and finally got to cuddle granddaughter number two.

"Isla struggled with her apnea, and had a multitude of tests to try to find out exactly what was going on, including brain scans. We felt so helpless but as any new parents would we wanted the best for our little girl. Finally on 27th October, six weeks after her birth. Isla came home with a mobile heart monitor.

"No book (and I read them all) could have prepared us for all the emotional highs and lows of those first three months of Isla and Megan's life. To be honest I don't think it is something that can be put into words but in their bedroom we have a small, framed card that says it all:

'When I count my blessings, I count you twice'."

I stayed in Houston for over a week but returned with Gary that Christmas, and Vicky joined us there too. She had recently moved from Ayr in Scotland to Phoenix, Arizona, where she sold corporate facilities and rooms at a vast, luxury resort hotel called The Phoenician. We spent an extra special family Christmas in Texas.

All too soon I had to return to the Channel Islands, and Guernsey in particular, where I had recently purchased two large properties. I had also bought The Bella Luce Hotel on the island.

The Bella was originally constructed as a Norman manorhouse (parts of the granite building date back to the 12th century), though the residence has been a hotel since the 1940s. The Bella Luce, nestled at the end of narrow country lanes at the top of a quiet valley, was extremely attractive on the outside, having been built from the pretty local pink granite. The interior was suffering from age and neglect.

Despite this, I was captivated by its charm from the outset. A lane meanders from the hotel down to Moulin Huet bay, a tiny gem of a beach surrounded by picturesque cliffs that the famed artist, Pierre-Auguste Renoir captured in a series of fifteen paintings. This was also the favourite picnic spot of Victor Hugo, the French author and poet who lived in exile on the island.

My partner in the venture was David Rondel, who oversaw the design and eight-month refurbishment of the hotel. We were both determined to honour the building's heritage, while adding modern essentials such as drainage, new electrics and plumbing, and replacing the roof, some windows and adding a new kitchen and bar.

The cost of it all was mammoth, but we were both proud of the end result. The hotel was transformed into a work of art. David deserves all the credit.

The Bella Luce is a member of Britain's Finest Hotels and the group of Small Luxury Hotels of the World. By the time it re-opened the refurbishment costs had escalated to such an extent that I had to bring in another partner to the venture. Luke Wheadon, whose family had once owned and lived in the original manor house, became involved in the day-to-day running of the business.

All was going well, or so I thought, in 2008. My property portfolio was building up and by that time I had bought and sold over £30million worth of houses, flats and commercial premises. I was generally enjoying life. I took my girlfriend at the time, Louise, to stay at L'Hermitage in Monte Carlo. I bumped into my old friends Alan and Wendy Murphy again. They invited us to attend a charity dinner where Trevor McDonald was guest speaker.

However, little did I realise the scale of the impending financial crisis that was gathering on the world's horizon. Certainly the property market was slowing down and there were cash flow problems at The Bella Luce. Having survived so many crises, I tried to remain positive.

In the summer of 2009 a tall, imposing man with silver hair walked into The Bella and said he was looking for an intimate, comfortable hotel. He explained that he had already visited several hotels but hadn't yet found something to suit him. I arranged for the impressive gent to be shown around. He loved The Bella Luce.

My guest was Roddie Fleming, the nephew of James Bond creator Ian. We enjoyed many evenings together, having supper at his favourite table beside the roaring fire. Apart from the James Bond stories, I was intrigued to learn all about his multi-billion pound banking business.

One day I casually mentioned an amazing super yacht, Le Grand Bleu, which I had recently seen moored off the Isle of Wight.

'Would you like to meet the man who owns it?' Roddie asked.

'I'd love to,' I replied eagerly.

'Then I'll arrange a meeting in London. The yacht is owned by Eugene Shvidler. He received the yacht as a present from Roman Abramovich.'

And so, a short time later, I was invited to lunch at

a restaurant in London where Roddie introduced me to Eugene. He was immaculately dressed and groomed and seemed delighted that I had shown such an interest in his yacht,

We also talked about Chateau Thénac, a vineyard in the heart of the Périgord region of France that he had recently purchased and renovated. After lunch, we all walked down to a cigar shop close to the Ritz Hotel where we sat chatting in the smoking room at the back of the shop. He was interested in my various business interests over the years and we spoke about promoting his wine through my hotel.

We met up again briefly in Guernsey, when Eugene had his jet diverted to the airport, much to the annoyance of his fellow directors. They had to hang around the hangar, while Roddie, Eugene and I had a meeting in the terminal building to discuss promoting Chateau Thénac and Le Grand Bleu through The Bella Luce. Nothing came from those talks, although the hotel did purchase a few cases of wine from his vineyard.

Since our time together at the Bella Luce, Roddie has shown himself to be a truly supportive friend. We meet up from time to time and it is always a pleasure to be with him and be entertained with his anecdotes.

By 2009 large cracks began to appear in my business. It was becoming increasingly difficult to get sufficient cash flowing through my various ventures.

Determined to put my problems to one side, at least for a few days, that Christmas I flew up to Inverness, hired a car and drove over to the Isle of Skye. Louisa and Keith owned a cottage with incredible views over the majestic snowbound forests and mountains. Being there with my family was so relaxing after the business strains of the past few months and helped to soothe my spirit. I returned to Guernsey where I spent New Year's Eve at The Bella Luce with Roddie Fleming and Luke Wheadon, amongst others. But certainly, as the calendar turned in 2010, I was filled with concern about the future.

Three weeks later, at my regular hospital check-up, my blood test showed that the platelet count had fallen under the normal figure of 200. My myelofibrosis was on its way back. Perhaps naively, I had thought that one bone marrow transplant would sort me out for life. As time progressed, so did the illness until my platelet count had fallen to 8. I was once again requiring regular transfusions.

Gary's sixtieth birthday in March at least provided a good distraction from all of my problems. We joined a group of his friends at Incognito, a restaurant in the heart of London's theatreland.

Not long after this, the oncologists at St George's Hospital decided that they would perform a lymphocyte donation from Axel, with the hope that the donor cells would trigger Axel's bone marrow cells in my body. When I emailed Axel he was true to his word and, without hesitation, agreed to being my donor once more. He immediately made an appointment with DKMS to have his lymphocyte cells harvested.

On the day of the harvest, 13 July 2010, Axel attended the clinic, where he switched off his mobile phone and underwent the four-and-a-half hour procedure. Unknown to him, his wife Stephanie had gone into premature labour at exactly the same time. She had an emergency caesarean procedure, giving birth to their daughter two months early.

Axel was in total shock after his day of high drama. I was touched to receive an e-mail, wishing me well, despite the fact that I had caused him to miss the birth of his daughter.

His e-mail said: "*The day started to be quite normal, like any of the others that week. All was perfect between me and my wife Stephanie. We were happily expecting our first child – Stephanie was seven months pregnant. I checked my emails and saw one from Eric* in England, whose life I had saved with my stem cells in September 2004. I was privileged to meet him personally in 2006. Since then we have spent two exciting holidays together and now feel bound by a great friendship.

I was surprised by that e-mail. Eric was asking me once more to donate lymphocytes, since his last health check had shown irregularities. I immediately knew that I would want to help my friend again. I quickly made an appointment with DKMS where they received recent notice from Eric's consultants about another urgent donation – for a cell harvest to be taken at a clinic in Hameln.

On 13 July 2010, all was organised and I made way to Hameln where I was most warmly greeted – due to a minor concern, my wife had been transferred into a hospital for observation the day before, but we had no serious worries. Once I arrived in Hameln I switched off my mobile phone. At that time my wife started with heavy bleeding. Stephanie decided not to let me know about her predicament so as not to endanger the harvest of Eric's so important cells. Shortly afterwards her situation changed dramatically.

I knew absolutely nothing of it all. While I felt calm and wired up to various pieces of apparatus for the cell donation, a medical team eighty kilometres away decided to start birth procedures. Our child was helped into the world by caesarean section, two months premature.

After four and a half hours I had given enough cells. I felt hungry and made my way to the in-house canteen to have lunch. At that stage our daughter was already three hours into this world and I was still completely clueless.

I left the hospital feeling elated that I had helped Eric and directed myself towards visiting my wife. My mobile was still switched off. And why not, since I would soon be in yet another clinic. The news which awaited me there hit me totally unprepared. My daughter had been born! It felt absolutely beautiful. But I was also in a bit of a shock and felt very sorry for my wife. It had always been my wish to be by her side at the birth of our first child. To Stephanie, it was comforting that, like her, I had given *someone the chance to live at exactly the same time on the same hot day in July.*

That evening I wrote an email to Eric feeling relieved and happy, giving him my report of this incredible day. Later he told me that it had moved him to tears. He felt very unimaginably sorry that I had not been able to be present at the birth of my daughter.

From now there will be another person, also connected through a fine bond with Eric. Our little Lena will be able to entertain in future with a story about her father who has helped another man to live the same day she was born. I am already looking forward to introducing her soon to my English big brother, Eric"

Axel's cells arrived at St George's, frozen in a special container and were then defrosted in my room, before I received them by drip into my bloodstream.

However, despite this procedure, the hoped-for improvement in my cell count was not to be. So the transfusions continued and the drugs to reduce my iron levels commenced again. I was back in the old pre-transplant medical routine that I hoped to leave behind.

I accepted the situation and continued with my visits to St George's and the oncology clinic at the General Hospital in St Helier, between making the most of my very comfortable apartment at the harbour,

My family was clearly upset with this setback in my health but, as ever, they were most supportive. They appreciated how strong I had been for the bone marrow transplant and knew I would cope well when the time came again. Meanwhile, I had plenty to keep me busy work-wise as I struggled to make my various business projects stack up financially.

For my sixtieth birthday the following March, my extended family came to spend a few days with me at The Bella Luce. All the fires were lit against the late winter weather and we enjoyed a procession of fine meals with other friends. We loved bracing walks on the beaches and cliffs nearby before retreating back into the cosy hotel.

It was certainly the highlight of the year for me, and also something of a marker. Despite all the problems in my business, and the fact that I was having blood transfusions again, I felt grateful to be alive.

By early 2012, property prices had fallen so much that I was in danger of losing everything. For example one of my apartments lost a third of its value, virtually overnight. As the months passed I went through stages of denial and anger as I mentally and emotionally prepared myself for losing everything. Eventually I came to a place of acceptance.

And so in January 2013, my businesses had reached what I felt was an irretrievable position. I approached my solicitor to begin the process of voluntary bankruptcy with the Viscount's Department of the States of Jersey. This is the administrative office of the Jersey Courts and States Assembly.

It was a poignant time. I had transacted over eighty properties with my solicitor in Jersey alone since my return to the island; however, by then I had already gone through the bankruptcy in my head and left my possessions behind.

The process of going bankrupt on the island is called Désastre, and at the end of January I was declared en Désastre.

I dealt with a lady at the Viscount's Department, and she managed to make the whole process more palatable than I ever could have imagined. For that, I was immensely grateful.

I was grateful to Eric and Valerie Morgan, who were so supportive at this time. We had become friends after viewing one of their properties on the island. Eric and I would talk for hours about our lives and adventures, while Valerie attended to all our needs. Friends for life – and there is definitely a book in Eric Morgan!

The news obviously spread through all my contacts on Jersey like wildfire, as the island is so small. It was interesting to find out who really cared about me, while many turned their backs. They were either embarrassed or feared that I would ask for a loan. Chris Brien certainly showed himself to be a true friend, as did Roddie Fleming, and my family were there for me, as always.

I slowly sorted out my affairs, putting some of my possessions into storage, before moving out of my apartment with vital personal items. Of course, on the surface it appeared to be a catastrophe, but in truth we never really own anything. We are, at best, guardians of possessions for a while. In addition, the process had taught me a great deal about what really matters in life.

The other advantage of the situation was that, without the stress involved in running an unravelling business, I was able to concentrate on my health. I had to be in the best possible shape for my next transplant. I was also able to spend more time with my family.

There was no point in wasting any time or energy, dwelling over my material losses. I had very little material possessions left.

Scarlett and the other children flashed through my mind. They had much less than me. All they possessed: a collection of rags and a few bags of rice.

And yet they always retained their dignity.

A lesson for us all.

CHAPTER FIFTEEN

My Fight for Survival

August 7th 2014. Day sixteen at St George's Hospital

And so here I am at St George's Hospital, London, on August 7th 2014. The day is much the same as yesterday; the only difference is that some of my hair is falling out. This is a trivial matter really, and I shall probably soon shave it all off.

The doctors are expecting white cells to begin showing in my blood tests at some point soon. And, as I have done every day since my admission, I focus my attention on a positive end result for my transplant.

With all that I have with me I'm certainly not bored or lonely, especially as Vicky, Louisa, Gary and David have all stayed in constant contact.

August 8th 2014

The morning passes easily in the pattern of four-hourly checks, a blood test and regular meals and medication that I've become so used to. I am genuinely feeling well, if very tired.

Each day I wait for Mickey Koh, the consultant haematologist, to tell me that the neutrophils and white cells are on the move. This would be the first sign of a successful outcome to my bone marrow transplant. I decide not to ask, but be patient.

So no news today on my neutrophils; perhaps tomorrow, I think, as I take my sleeping pill for the night.

August 9th 2014

I spend the morning quietly passing the time and then Mickey arrives. Is this the day, I wonder? He says I am doing extremely well and he expects to see my neutrophils come up by Monday, in two days' time. It's great news and I'm really excited and appreciate the update and information. Nevertheless, I keep thinking that perhaps there will be neutrophils in the blood test tomorrow. As ever, I think only about a positive outcome.

August 10th 2014

The clumps of hair on my pillow this morning tell me that this is the day to shave my head! Aside from that, I eat quite well – and am certainly pleased, as are the staff, that my weight has dropped by just two kilos since my admission.

It is now ten days since my transplant and, as the nurses take my blood for testing, I wonder if today will bring good news. As the day passes I reflect on my life before and after my first bone marrow transplant. There is so much history from over the years and I realise that my chance to create more memories all lies within my bone marrow.

No news from the haematology department today. I receive one of the regular calls from Valerie, and she passes me on to Eric. Just what I need. He asks me how I am feeling, and then we start talking business as we usually do. I must damp down my impatience, and mid-evening I take a sleeping pill to help accelerate the hours. Perhaps the good news will come tomorrow.

August 11th 2014

I wake pleased to put another night behind me and routine prevails with blood checks, pills, a shower and getting dressed for the day. I recall my last transplant and the moment the specialist came in and told me that my neutrophils had risen past zero for the first time. I remember being overwhelmed with relief. I drink my tea and remember the fifteen kilo weight-loss and intense sickness during the transplant in 2004. I reflect once more on how improved the procedure has become.

Breakfast over, I sit in my chair listening to music and at around 11.30 a.m. Mickey Koh walks in with a smile. 'How are you today?' he asks.

'Great! Just waiting for your visit to bring me some news!'

'Then you have it – your neutrophils are now showing at .1 – you are on your way!'

'You've been a good patient, so we will see a steady improvement over the next days. The result could not be better.'

I feel really emotional. A neutrophils count of .1 might not sound high, but coming from a count of zero their presence in my blood means that the transplant is starting to engraft.

I sit contemplating my good fortune. Yet another chance at life and all thanks to Axel Drewes, the DKMS team in Germany, the staff at the hospital in Dresden, the medical couriers, and of course all the doctors, nurses, consultants and other specialists here in the Ruth Myles Unit at St George's Hospital. Everyone has done everything necessary, day and night, to keep me alive and take me through this procedure. I have now reached the other side of the metaphorical gorge which I left twenty days ago. And I am smiling.

I text Axel with the news and then call my daughters and brothers, who are all thrilled and there are tears between us all. I also call every friend I can think of.

Finally, I settle down to relax. I listen to the two songs that I chose to encourage me through the transplant, Martina McBride's, In My Daughter's Eyes and Whitney Houston's One Moment in Time. The songs are beautiful and all is well now.

August 12th 2014

I wake excited and continue to write notes for my daily journal and call or text a few other people to pass on my good news. Later in the morning, my blood test result shows that the neutrophils count has risen to .3! My elation keeps growing and I thank each member of hospital staff who comes through my door. Their commitment to their job is impressive, as is that of the staff at Anthony Nolan, DKMS in Germany and their counterpart in the UK, Delete Blood Cancer. These organisations are doing profound work and are very dear to my heart.

For the first time since my admission, I allow myself to think of future plans. I will take as long as I need to fully recuperate and then decide on my next step in the adventure of life. Seeing more of my family, as well as taking the time to enjoy nature and its multitude of colours, is all that I truly desire.

Time is speeding up again, and Suzanne Ruggles comes to see me. She is thrilled. We talk about the Full Circle Fund and their work, and how much I have appreciated their efforts. We discuss my three reflexology sessions a week. We also talk about the value of living in the moment and letting the past go, and not worrying too much about tomorrow. The news about my improving health has filtered through to the day unit at the front of the ward. Huriye, one of the day unit patients, gives me the thumbs up at my window. She scuttles off to tell Gordon, another day patient who shares our wild sense of humour. We have caused uproar with all of our jokes and nonsense in the Day Unit.

August 13ᵗʰ 2014

It is Wednesday today, three weeks after my admission. I eat a breakfast of toast and a banana. Soon after 7.30 a.m. a blood sample is taken from the line in my chest. The progression upwards in my neutrophils count over the last two days is a key sign that all is going well. I spend the morning feeling excited at what the result will be today and am more than happy when the duty doctor comes just before noon to tell me neutrophils are .7 and my white blood cell count is 1.1.

As each reading improves, so does the feeling within my body: the nausea is abating and my strength slowly returning, though I realise I still have a long way to go. However, I am now able to look forward in my life. For the last four years I have lived with a blood count of between 7 and 8 – when 15 is the norm for men. Before long I will be producing blood products from 100% of Axel's stem cells, and that thought is uppermost in my mind. In the meantime all of my blood chemistry is looking excellent.

I receive wonderfully supportive messages from Axel, and my admiration for him could not be greater, although that's hard to convey adequately by text. The love from my family is clear in their words and faces that I see on screen.

I absorb it all gratefully, and appreciate the good wishes from friends and family. In particular Claire James and Suzanne Ruggles have been in touch daily to lift my spirits.

New technology has made a huge difference in making the isolation room a less lonely place than it was ten years ago.

August 14th 2014

I have had some pretty wild dreams with all the drugs I have been taking, though I realise that's all a part of the process towards my eventual discharge and rehabilitation.

As the routine continues I think of Louisa's twin daughters who will be seven in exactly a month – another reminder of how time appears to speed along. My thoughts also turn to Vicky who is now back in Aberdeen and preparing for her wedding in April 2015. Both of my daughters are happy and settled; that is wonderful for me, as other parents will appreciate.

The figures for my blood count arrive. The white cells are now 2.8 and the neutrophils 1.9; everyone is pleased with my progress, especially the patient. The rise in quick succession is a testament to Axel's good health. I text with the continuing good results and he replies with equal excitement.

I listen to some calming music in the afternoon and, after tea, take my pills and go to sleep at 7.30 p.m. The treatment has taken its toll on my body and I feel weak and tired by the end of the day. Time to rest and repair.

August 15th 2014

It's Friday today, and I decide to spend the time watching all the activity through the large internal window: the day is shorter if you make a plan. The corridor is generally busy with comings and goings from the day unit as well as the four other isolation rooms. I feel as though I'm in a zoo watching it all, but of course I'm the one who's being observed and have been in this isolation room now for just over three weeks.

The ever-smiling tea lady appears regularly throughout the day at the window like an actor making a stage entrance, bringing tea or coffee and my allocated packet of biscuits. As I can't hear her – and vice versa – I sign my request through the glass before she brings in my drink and, more often than not, two packets of biscuits. Breakfast, lunch and dinner appear outside the window in the same way, although the procedure quells your appetite and the feeling of nausea generally prevails over food. I have no taste or sense of smell.

Later in the day I receive confirmation that my white cells are now 4.3 and my neutrophils 3.2, which is another surprisingly good improvement on yesterday's figures.

I go to sleep while it's still light – another day behind me.

August 16th 2014

I wake early and lie on my bed just thinking about sleeping some more, but the hospital routine has a rhythm which thwarts that desire. Another obstacle to sleep is the line from my chest, hooked up to a drug which prevents my blood clotting. I've been attached to the line 24/7 since my admission. Sometimes visits to the bathroom have the feel of an assault course with this apparatus by my side; nevertheless it has probably helped to save my life, so I have resigned myself to its presence.

The day stretches as I'm feeling nauseous again and I struggle to settle and concentrate on anything. I flick through the TV channels looking for nature programmes or Grand Designs, which I always enjoy – and look forward to the next Grand Prix, a week away.

I fall asleep for three hours and when I wake I'm given my blood readings. I'm disappointed to learn that they have slipped to 4.1 for the white cells and 2.7 for the neutrophils, although I'm assured that this is normal and there is nothing to worry about.

Come the evening I'm still feeling tired and restless when Louisa and my granddaughters call me on Face Time, which lifts my mood considerably and distracts me from my nausea. This is a timely reminder about how you can change your state of mind, if you choose to, and prompts me to chat more to the hospital staff and escape my thoughts for a while. Nevertheless, I take a pill to get to sleep early yet again.

August 17th 2014

After a familiar morning I receive my blood results. To my mind, they show a significant drop – to 3.2 for white blood cells and 1.9 for neutrophils. The experts maintain this is normal, and the numbers will soon come up again.

I'm reassured by their opinion, accept the situation, and ask when they think I might be discharged: perhaps sometime later this coming week if all goes well, I'm told. This cheers me up as I'm looking forward to doing simple things such as going for a walk, albeit I feel weak and unsteady on my feet.

Enlivened, I try to focus on my puzzle. I've made little progress as my concentration still drifts all too easily. Music and TV are easier escapes as I can curl in my bed or chair and rest my body and head while no effort or thought is required. Still, I feel remarkably better than after my transplant in 2004, when I was in hospital for thirty-three days. I am now only two kilos lighter than my admission weight and feeling better in mind and body.

I allow my thoughts to wander to later in the year and Christmas, as my brand new life opens up before me. As I head to sleep, I am again full of gratitude for my progress and speed of recovery.

August 18ᵗʰ 2014

It is Monday morning and the doctors, consultants and senior nurses do their rounds to fully appraise and check over each patient. I ask a few questions, the most paramount of which is: when will I be released to go home?

'Looking at your results of white cells at 3.1 and neutrophils at 1.9, probably tomorrow and if not on Wednesday,' answers Mickey Koh.

The staff are all thrilled with my progress. I'm excited to hear about my impending release and thank everyone for their efforts and support. I could not have higher praise for all these professionals who have shown the utmost care and dedication. They've taken me to the brink of life and then brought me back to good health, all within such a short space of time. I know I'm privileged to be in such excellent hands.

When they leave the room it takes some strength to resist the urge to start packing, as I decide to wait until I have a definite departure date. Instead I make some Face Time calls and send texts to keep my friends and family updated.

August 19ᵗʰ 2014

After I receive my blood results I am told that I can go home at some stage tomorrow. A feeling of absolute relief washes over me. I can see who I want, when I want. I can go for walks again, see trees and flowers and everything else that nature has to offer. I have choices again.

Axel and his family have a special place in my heart. Axel is the only person who could have saved my life as a donor. I have enduring gratitude to DKMS, Delete Blood Cancer UK and Anthony Nolan. My new life is so close that I can almost feel it.

Axel sent me the following email describing his journey as a donor:

"When DKMS called me in 2004 to ask me to donate stem cells I was very excited about what would happen over the next few weeks. When I had my check-up and made the donation I was in good hands the whole time. The doctors and nurses were very nice and explained what was happening at every stage. After the donation I wondered about the person who was receiving my stem cells: where he/she lived; how old they were; and many other questions. Later on I learned that I had helped a man from the UK. I never felt like a hero, but it was great to know that I had helped someone in need. I always said that I would make another donation if someone needed it, but I never expected that to be in both 2010 and 2014 for Eric again. When we first met in Marbella in 2006 we spent a lot of time talking together and Eric told me many things about his illness. After that I understood what a difficult time Eric had before he got my stem cells. For me it was just a little thing to donate stem cells, but for Eric it is the chance of a second life. Thanks to all the people who have helped make Eric healthy again. Best wishes, my friend, and all the best for your new life."

August 20th 2014. The final day

It is my final day in the isolation room, exactly four weeks from my admission to the Ruth Myles Unit. It has been an incredible journey of mind and body, albeit I know I still have a long way to go in my recovery. Undoubtedly the most difficult part of that process is now over.

I pack slowly, to savour completing this stage of the process. There's my case of clothes, my briefcase with various papers and my diary and iPad inside, plus another small bag with my books, puzzles and photos and other personal items. After that, I'm ready to go and call Gary to let him know that my final medication is being written up and sent to the pharmacy. I ask him to come at around 3.30 p.m. He arrives just as I receive two large bags of drugs with their instructions.

Opening the door of the isolation room I am unsteady on my feet but determined to walk out of the ward and the hospital, and not be wheeled out as I was ten years ago. I walk slowly down the corridor with Gary, past the day unit and entrance to the lifts.

We wait a while for the lift to come and then it takes us to the ground floor and the long corridor to the car park.

I see the doors in the distance and, although I'm unsteady to say the least, I feel that I am being pulled towards them.

As I approach the doors I feel a sense of exhilaration. I have achieved all that I set out to do. I manage to push open one of the doors and walk out the hospital unaided. I gasp as the first fresh air for a month fills my lungs.

I take a brief look back and reflect on my six decades. My disastrous spell at boarding school; the rearing Gale Force 12 in the North Sea; making my first million; the terror at Orly Airport; the search for Stalin's gold; my adventures in America; my escapades with Sue in Liberia; the moment my logging company collapsed before my eyes; the dramatic escape from a civil war; and the joy of fatherhood as well as becoming a grandad and uncle.

I walk on and turn my head again. I remember Axel; I think about Siafa; I recall with disgust my brutal interrogators.

A timeline runs through my head as I walk across the car park and stare straight ahead. I feel so fortunate to be given yet another chance in life.

I have no idea how long I will survive after my new transplant. Every day I live and breathe, I will always remember a group of African children and a thoughtful, deep, silent little girl I called Scarlett.

Axel gave me life in a bag, and his total commitment. Scarlett gave me my freedom.

They will never leave my thoughts.

Acknowledgements

To everyone who has been part of my life. I would like to say again: 'In the moment of something that appears so awful are the seeds of something wonderful. The only problem is – will you recognise that moment when it arrives?'

My heart-felt thanks go to the multi-disciplinary team involved in my stem cell transplant at St George's Hospital: Mickey Koh, my transplant consultant and his fellow team of consultants who ensured my 24-hour cover; the specialist registrars and ward-based doctors; clinical transplant fellow; transplant co-coordinator; Apheresis team for stem cell collection; ward nurses; Day Unit nurses; stem cell processing scientists; pharmacist; dietician; physiotherapy/occupational therapy staff; Quality Manager; Data Manager; Medical Secretaries.

In addition, I would like to thank the following supporting disciplines:

Laboratory staff and Blood Bank Officers; Infectious Disease and Microbiology Team; Intensive Care Unit; Essential Specialities Cardiology; Respiratory Medicine; Liver Specialists; Renal Team; Radiology and Access to scans/ imaging; Hospital Estates who maintain the air flow filtration George's Hospital; and the Full Circle Fund.

I am grateful to my friend and author Caroline J. Christensen for her guidance and invaluable observations with this book. I am indebted to author and copy editor David Meikle for his insight, advice and prose, as well as his unique flair for structure and storytelling.

I wish to thank Lisa Le Gresley for being my friend, introducing me to Caroline J. Christensen and for a personal nudge in getting me to finally complete the book.

And, having met journalist Neil Hyde at The Bella Luce in Guernsey, a thank you for his introduction to author David Meikle.

Afterword by Roddie Fleming, nephew of James Bond creator Ian Fleming

I first met Eric through his ownership of the Bella Luce Hotel in Guernsey. I had arrived to spend some months there and, after a quick tour of all the major hotels, I quickly settled for the Bella.

It had such a comfortable and welcoming atmosphere, proving quite irresistible on first acquaintance. Not only was it a lap of luxury but also it sported a kitchen of great and fattening talent. Many a pound was put on for a good cause at the Bella. But then, with all the abundance of rich cream from the Guernsey udders and the multitude of fresh fish from the strong currents of the Channel seas, the very word 'diet' has faded from the Islanders' lexicon.

The islands sported a large German garrison during the years of the War – and no surprises there. The lure of days on the Eastern Front must have paled,

There is a hymn which ends with the line "still small voice of calm". I always think that Eric must have been the inspiration for this. For quiet courage, quiet conviction, quiet humour – for the 'quiet word', Eric is the master.

As Andrew Devonshire said: "Never underestimate the power of silence."

Anthony Nolan Afterword

Anthony Nolan currently need more young men aged 16-30 to sign up, as they are most likely to be chosen to donate but make up only 14% of the register. They also urgently need people from Black, Asian and other Ethnic Minority backgrounds, as they are currently under-represented on the register.

People who sign on to the Anthony Nolan register remain there until they are sixty years old. However, because of thousands of tissue types out there, only one in a thousand people who join the register actually get a call asking them to donate. There is no cost at all to join the register or to donate bone marrow or stem cells; however, it costs Anthony Nolan around £100 to recruit and type tissue their potentially lifesaving donors. The charity relies on the generosity of people who give money to support their work.

Liberia Factfile

Portuguese explorers established contacts with Liberia as early as 1461 and named the area 'Grain Coast' because of the abundance of grains of Melegueta Pepper.

In 1663 the British installed trading posts in the Grain Coast, but the Dutch destroyed them a year later. There were no further reports of European settlements along the Grain Coast until the arrival of freed slaves in the early 1800s.

Liberia, meaning 'land of the free', was founded by freed slaves from the United States in 1820. These freed slaves, called Americo-Liberians, first arrived and established a settlement in Christopolis, now Monrovia (named after U.S. president James Monroe) on 6 February 1820. This group of eighty-six immigrants formed the nucleus of the settler population of the Republic of Liberia.

Thousands of freed slaves arrived from America, culminating in a Declaration of Independence on 26 July, 1847 of the Republic of Liberia.

In 1862, the American President, Abraham Lincoln, extended official recognition to Liberia.

In 1865, more than three hundred immigrants from Barbados joined the small number of African Americans coming to Liberia after the American Civil War.

Liberia's history until 1980 was largely peaceful. Long after independence, the Republic of Liberia was a one-party state ruled by the Americo-Liberian dominated True Whig Party (TWP). Joseph Jenkins Roberts, who was born and raised in America, became Liberia's first president.

On 12 April 1980 Liberian Master Sergeant Samuel K Doe, from the Krahn ethnic group, seized power in a coup d'état. Doe's forces executed President William R. Tolbert and several officials of his government, who were mostly of Americo-Liberian descent. As result, 133 years of Americo-Liberian political domination ended with the formation of the People's Redemption Council (PRC).

Political parties remained banned until 1984. Elections were held on 15 October of that year in which Doe's National Redemption Party was declared victorious. The elections were characterised by widespread fraud and rigging. The period after the elections saw increased human rights abuses, corruption and ethnic tensions.

On 12 November 1985, former army Commander General Thomas Quiwonkpa invaded Liberia by way of neighbouring Sierra Leone and almost succeeded in toppling the government of Samuel Doe. The Armed Forces of Liberia repelled Quiwonkpa's attack and executed him in Monrovia.

On 24 December, 1989, a small band of rebels led by Doe's former procurement chief, Charles Taylor, invaded Liberia from the Ivory Coast. Taylor and his National Patriotic Front rebels rapidly gained the support of Liberians because of the repressive nature of Samuel Doe and his government.

The Liberian Civil war, which was one of the bloodiest, claimed the lives of more than 200,000 Liberians and further displaced a million others into refugee camps in neighbouring countries. The Economic Community of West African States intervened and succeeded in preventing Charles Taylor from Capturing Monrovia.

Prince Johnson, who had been a member of Taylor's National Patriotic Front, broke away because of policy differences. Johnson's forces captured and killed Doe on 9 September, 1990.

In April 2012, former president Charles Taylor was found guilty of war crimes. He was sentenced to fifty years in jail, to be served in Britain.

Tribute to the Slaves

Throughout the book I have discussed Liberia's crucial place in history and the relocation of freed slaves.

William Wilberforce, one of the greatest reformers in history, regarded slavery as a crime. He said that all Englishmen were responsible, and the practice must come to an end. In 1814 Wilberforce and his friends gathered one million signatures, a tenth of the population, in 800 petitions and delivered them to the House of Commons.

The Abolition of the Slave Trade Act had been passed in 1807 – with nothing done to free the existing slaves in the British Empire.

Eventually in 1833 Parliament passed the second reading of the Slave Emancipation Act, ensuring the end of slavery in the British Empire. Three days later, Wilberforce died.

This meant that hundreds of thousands of Africans, who were then the legal property of Britain's slave owners, were freed. However, the Act stated that there should be financial compensation for the owners of those slaves, by the British taxpayer. This would allow for the loss of the slave owners' property!

The Compensation Commission was established to evaluate and administer the claims of the slave owners.

After all the claims had been assessed, the staggering amount of £20 million in compensation was paid to the slave owners. This unbelievable sum was 40% of the total government expenditure in 1834.

To put the amount of compensation in perspective, it would be the equivalent of £16.5 billion today.

Enormous amounts of money were passed down through

families, and prominent people in the United Kingdom have benefited, through their ancestors, from the slave trade.

The slaves, of course, received nothing. To add insult to injury, they were compelled to provide more than 40 hours of unpaid labour each week. This continued for four years after their so-called 'liberation'.

Only children under six years old were freed immediately. Everyone else was ordered to work those extra hours a week for nothing until 1840 – although they did receive free board and lodgings! Amidst howls of protests, the deadline was brought forward to 1838. Finally, 700,000 slaves in the West Indies were freed along with 40,000 in South Africa and 20,000 in Mauritius.

The slave owners moved into other more constructive and still profitable pursuits. They shaped Britain's future in railways, shipping, banking and industry.

All of those downtrodden, abused slaves throughout the British Empire gave everything and received so little.

They paid for their liberation with blood, sweat and tears. Many paid with their lives.